Are You Ready to Improve Diabetes Care?

Congratulations—you are among 100,000 physicians, physician assistants, nurse practitioners, nurses, and diabetes educators/dietitians who have received a complimentary copy of the *ACP Diabetes Care Guide*. Produced by the editors of the Medical Knowledge Self-Assessment Program® (MKSAP®), the leading source of self-assessment education in internal medicine, the Diabetes Care Guide will help you provide better care across multidisciplinary lines.

You will find the text inside conversational yet authoritative, presenting state-of-the-art practices and important information based on best evidence. A committee of leading experts has worked hard to create a book that is accessible, featuring a flexible binding that allows you to flip to a helpful page or two and make copies for other members of your care team. The book includes special tools for the health-care team as well as for patients. Tools designated *For Better Practice* facilitate effective team collaboration and education. Tools designated *For Better Health* are for handing out to patients to improve patient education and self-care, with advice on how to manage medications, exercise, diet, lifestyle changes, and other issues of importance.

The companion CD-ROM inside this book allows you to test your knowledge by answering 81 multiple-choice questions modeled after the questions used for internal medicine's certifying examination. By completing the test and submitting it online, you can qualify for any of the following:

- 15 *AMA PRA Category 1 Credits*™ if you are a physician

- 15 non-physician Continuing Medical Education credits if you are a physician assistant, as authorized under AMA guidelines
- 15 Continuing Education credits if you are a nurse practitioner or nurse
- 15 Continuing Professional Education credits if you are a dietitian

Although the continuing education credits and the Care Guide are free of charge, significant resources were needed to develop the program, which was underwritten by an unrestricted educational grant from Novo Nordisk. The Care Guide is part of the ACP Diabetes Initiative, which also includes the ACP Diabetes Portal (http://diabetes.acponline.org) and other activities to promote improved diabetes care. (Information on the initiative is available at http://www.acponline.org/college/pressroom/diab_care.htm.)

As you will read, many experts believe medical practices should use multidisciplinary team–based models of care to overcome barriers that block improved outcomes for patients with diabetes. Completion of this program will help to prepare you to adopt such a model in your practice. We hope you take advantage of this important opportunity. Please share this resource with other members of your team and use it to develop a plan for success in your health care setting.

Vincenza Snow, MD, FACP
Clinical Director
Diabetes Initiative Program
American College of Physicians

ACP Diabetes Care Guide
A Team-Based Practice Manual and Self-Assessment Program

American College of Physicians, Philadelphia, Pennsylvania

ISBN: 978-1-930513-91-4

Printed in the United States of America.

For information on this program, call 800-523-1546, extension 2600.

Educational Disclaimer

The editors and publisher of *ACP Diabetes Care Guide: A Team-Based Practice Manual and Self-Assessment Program* recognize that the development of new material offers many opportunities for error. Despite our best efforts, some errors may persist in print. Drug dosage schedules are, we believe, accurate and in accordance with current standards. Readers are advised, however, to ensure that the recommended dosages in this program concur with the information provided in the product information material. This is especially important in cases of new, infrequently used, or highly toxic drugs. Application of the information in the Guide in a professional situation remains the professional responsibility of the practitioner.

The primary purpose of the *ACP Diabetes Care Guide: A Team-Based Practice Manual and Self-Assessment Program* is educational. Information presented, as well as publications, technologies, products, and/or services discussed, is intended to inform subscribers about the knowledge, techniques, and experiences of the contributors. A diversity of professional opinion exists, and the views of the contributors are their own and not those of the ACP. Inclusion of any material in the Guide does not constitute endorsement or recommendation by the ACP. The ACP does not warrant the safety, reliability, accuracy, completeness or usefulness of and disclaims any and all liability for damages and claims that may result from the use of information, publications, technologies, products, and/or services discussed in this program.

Co-Editors

Martin J. Abrahamson, MD[2]
Medical Director
Joslin Diabetes Center
Associate Professor of Medicine
Harvard Medical School
Boston, Massachusetts

Mark Aronson, MD, FACP[2]
Vice Chairman for Quality
Department of Medicine
Beth Israel Deaconess Medical Center
Professor of Medicine
Harvard Medical School
Boston, Massachusetts

Contributors

Catherine Carver, MS, APRN, BC, CDE[1]
Director, Care & Education
Joslin Clinic
Boston, Massachusetts

Jody Dushay, MD[1]
Clinical Fellow in Endocrinology
Beth Israel Deaconess Medical Center
Boston, Massachusetts

Martha M. Funnell, MS, RN, CDE[2]
Co-Director, Behavioral, Clinical and Health Systems
  Intervention Core
Diabetes Research and Training Center
University of Michigan
Ann Arbor, Michigan

Jason L. Gaglia, MD[2]
Research Fellow
Joslin Diabetes Center
Instructor in Medicine
Beth Israel Deaconess Medical Center
Harvard Medical School
Boston, Massachusetts

Om Ganda, MD[2]
Associate Clinical Professor of Medicine
Harvard Medical School
Director, Lipid Clinic
Joslin Diabetes Center
Boston, Massachusetts

Michele Heisler, MD, MPA[1]
Assistant Professor/Research Scientist
Ann Arbor VA Center for Practice Management and
  Outcomes Research
VA Ann Arbor Health System
Department of Internal Medicine
University of Michigan Health System
Ann Arbor, Michigan

Lucy A. Levandoski, PA-C[2]
Clinical Diabetes Research Coordinator
Washington University School of Medicine
St. Louis, Missouri

Medha N. Munshi, MD[2]
Director, Joslin Geriatric Diabetes Clinic
Director, Outpatient Geriatric Programs
Beth Israel Deaconess Medical Center
Instructor, Harvard Medical School
Boston, Massuchusetts

Principal ACP Staff

*Senior Vice President, Medical Education
  and Publishing*
Steven Weinberger, MD, FACP[2]

Vice President, Medical Education and Publishing
D. Theresa Kanya, MBA[1]

Director, Self-Assessment Programs
Sean McKinney[1]

Managing Editor
Charles Rossi[1]

Senior Staff Editors
Becky Krumm[1]
Ellen M. McDonald, PhD[1]

Director, Clinical Programs and Quality of Care
Vincenza Snow, MD[1]

*Senior Research Associate, Research Planning
  and Evaluation*
Kevin Siddons, EdD[1]

Administrative Staff

Production Administrator
Sheila O'Steen

Program Administrator
Valerie Dangovetsky

Editorial Coordinators
Karen Williams
Katie Idell

---

[1]Has no relationships with any proprietary entity that provides health care goods or services, with the exception of nonprofit or government organizations and non–health care–related companies.

[2]Has disclosed relationship(s) with any proprietary entity that provides health care goods or services, with the exception of nonprofit or government organizations and non–health care–related companies.

Continuing Medical Education for Physicians

The American College of Physicians is accredited by the Accreditation Council for Continuing Medical Education (ACCME) to provide continuing medical education for physicians.

The American College of Physicians designates this educational activity for a maximum of 15 *AMA PRA Category 1 Credits*[TM]. Physicians should only claim credit commensurate with the extent of their participation in the activity.

The American Medical Association has determined that physicians not licensed in the United States who participate in this CME activity are eligible for *AMA PRA Category 1 Credit*[TM].

AMA PRA Category 1 Credit[TM] is available from April 13, 2007 to April 13, 2010.

Continuing Medical Education for Physician Assistants

The American Academy of Physician Assistants (AAPA) accepts *AMA PRA Category 1* credits from organizations accredited by the ACCME. The provider of this program, the American College of Physicians, is accredited by the ACCME and designates this educational activity for a maximum of 15 *AMA PRA Category 1 Credits*[TM]. Physician assistants should only claim credit commensurate with the extent of their participation in the activity.

AMA PRA Category 1 Credit[TM] is available from April 13, 2007 to April 13, 2010.

Continuing Education for Nurses and Nurse Practitioners

This continuing nursing education activity was approved for 15 contact hours by the PA State Nurses Association, an accredited approver by the American Nurses Credentialing Center's Commission on Accreditation.

CE credit is available from April 13, 2007 to April 13, 2009.

Continuing Professional Education for Dietitians

This continuing professional education activity was approved for 15 hours of credit by the American Association of Diabetes Educators.

CPE credit is available from April 13, 2007 to May 31, 2009.

Instructions for Earning CME, CE, and CPE Credit

To earn up to a maximum of 15 CME credits, read the program, answer 30% of the 81 multiple-choice questions on the CD-ROM correctly, submit your answers online, complete the required online program evaluation form at the end of the questions, and submit the form electronically. (Instructions are available on the CD-ROM.) The same instructions apply for those submitting for CE or CPE credits. You will gain access to an electronic certificate confirming the number of credits you have earned. Print out the certificate for your records. A record of your participation will be transferred via the Web to the American College of Physicians. As required, the College will retain records for 5 years for nurses, 6 years for physicians and physician assistants, and 7 years for dietitians. Note: You must submit completed tests *while online* to qualify for CME, CE, and CPE credits.

Objectives

After completing the *ACP Diabetes Care Guide*, you should be better able to achieve the following objectives:

1. Determine which aspects of diabetes care need to be improved in your medical practice.
2. Establish a care team for patients with diabetes.
3. Provide self-management education to patients with newly diagnosed diabetes.
4. Provide ongoing diabetes self-management support to patients with previously diagnosed diabetes.
5. Recognize the various types of diabetes.
6. Describe how to diagnose diabetes.
7. Determine who should be screened for diabetes.
8. Recognize when to screen for gestational diabetes.
9. Teach patients how to prevent diabetes.
10. Recommend meal planning for patients with diabetes.
11. Teach patients with diabetes how to increase their physical activity.
12. Teach patients how to self-monitor blood glucose levels.
13. Teach patients with diabetes how to take oral diabetes drugs.
14. Teach patients with diabetes how to use insulin.
15. Teach patients with diabetes how to use injectable drugs.
16. Teach patients with diabetes how to set weight loss goals.
17. Teach patients with diabetes the benefits of controlling hyperlipidemia.
18. Teach patients with diabetes the benefits of controlling hypertension.
19. Screen patients with diabetes for depression.
20. Screen patients with diabetes for cognitive dysfunction.
21. Teach patients with diabetes the risks of complications.
22. Teach patients with diabetes how to prevent diabetic retinopathy.
23. Screen patients with diabetes annually for microalbuminuria.
24. Implement foot examinations to prevent amputations associated with peripheral vascular disease (PVD) and diabetic foot ulcers.
25. Determine which coronary artery disease risk factors should be present in patients with diabetes to recommend cardiac stress testing.
26. Screen for neuropathies in patients with diabetes.
27. Teach women of childbearing age who have diabetes to care for their diabetes.
28. Monitor pregnant women with diabetes for retinopathy, nephropathy, neuropathy, cardiovascular disease, and hypertension.
29. Administer oral medications to elderly patients who have diabetes.
30. Teach elderly patients with diabetes and their families how these patients can avoid hypoglycemia.
31. Recognize which ethnic groups have a higher prevalence of type 2 diabetes, impaired glucose tolerance, and gestational diabetes than do white Americans.
32. Respond to emergencies that arise in diabetes care.
33. Provide hospital care for patients with diabetes.

Target Audience

- General internists and primary care physicians
- Endocrinologists seeking to improve multidisciplinary care of patients with diabetes
- Subspecialists who participate in the multidisciplinary care of patients with diabetes
- Residents of internal medicine
- Physician assistants
- Nurse practitioners
- Nurses
- Diabetes educators, including dietitians

Acknowledgments

The American College of Physicians gratefully acknowledges the special contributions to the development and production of the *ACP Diabetes Care Guide: A Team-Based Practice Manual and Self-Assessment Program* of Scott Thomas Hurd (Systems Analyst/Developer), Ricki Jo Kauffman (Senior Systems Analyst/Developer), and Elizabeth Swartz (Graphic Services Manager). The CD-ROM was developed within the American College of Physicians' Electronic Product Development department by Steven Spadt (Director), senior software developers Sean O'Donnell, Elijah Odumosu, and Brian Sweigard, and software developers Chris Forrest and

John McKnight. The College also wishes to acknowledge that many other persons, too numerous to mention, have contributed to the production of this program. Without their dedicated efforts, this program would not have been possible.

Commercial Support

This CME, CE, and CPE activity is underwritten by an unrestricted educational grant from Novo Nordisk. Approval of this continuing nursing education activity refers to recognition of the educational activity only and does not imply ANCCC Commission on Accreditation or PA Nurses approval or endorsement of any product.

Disclosure

It is the policy of the American College of Physicians (ACP) to ensure balance, independence, objectivity, and scientific rigor in all its educational activities. To this end, and consistent with the policies of the ACP and the Accreditation Council for Continuing Medical Education (ACCME), contributors to all ACP continuing medical education activities are required to disclose all financial relationships they have with proprietary entities producing health care goods or services, with the exception of nonprofit or government organizations and non–health care–related companies. Contributors are required to use generic names in the discussion of therapeutic options and are required to identify any unapproved, off-label, or investigative use of commercial products or devices. Where a trade name is used, all available trade names for the same product type are also included. If trade-name products manufactured by companies with whom they have relationships are discussed, contributors are asked to provide evidence-based citations in support of the discussion. The information is reviewed by the committee responsible for producing this text. If necessary, adjustments to topics or contributors' roles in content development are made to balance the discussion. Further, all readers of this text are asked to evaluate the content for evidence of commercial bias so that future decisions about content and contributors can be made in light of this information.

To resolve all conflicts and influences of vested interests, the ACP precluded members of the content creation committee from deciding on any content issues that involved generic or trade name products associated with proprietary entities with which those committee members had financial relationships. Contributors' disclosure information can be found with the list of contributors' names at the beginning of this book.

Contents

Introduction—A Call to Action

Why Team-Based Care of Patients with Diabetes Is So Important

One in every 14 Americans has diabetes, and another 40% of the population are at risk for developing the disease. Every year, diabetes accounts for more than 200,000 deaths, 82,000 amputations, and 44,400 new cases of end-stage renal disease and up to 24,000 new cases of blindness in the United States. Although proven strategies have been developed to identify and care for persons with diabetes, thus delaying the progression of the disease and reducing its complications, a serious gap exists between established recommendations and the actual care patients receive. Consider the following:

- Type 2 diabetes is undiagnosed in nearly 50% of persons with the disease.

- Approximately 58% of adults with diabetes have hemoglobin A1C levels that exceed the American Diabetes Association goal of less than 7%.

- In the National Health and Nutrition Examination Survey data from 1999–2000, only 7% of adults with diabetes achieved desired goals for glycemic control, blood pressure, and lipid level.

The barriers to providing optimal care are many and include socioeconomic factors such as access to preventive and specialty care, cost of physician visits and prescription drugs, and insurer payment policies. In addition, nonspecialists often feel ill-equipped—in terms of training, time, office staffing, and other aspects of practice—to provide the kind of ongoing, patient-centered care with intensive patient tracking and follow-up procedures that are now being recommended for patients with complicated chronic illnesses such as diabetes. The broad variety of practice settings where patients with diabetes receive care—from small general medicine clinics to large academic diabetes treatment centers—challenge the creation of an optimum, standardized approach to long-term management of this chronic, progressive disease.

Quality of Care Initiatives

Many organizations have developed guidelines to aid clinicians in their care of patients with diabetes. Indeed, so persuasive are the data on improved outcomes with tight glycemic, blood pressure, and lipid control that many insurers have adopted the National Committee for Quality Assurance (NCQA) HEDIS criteria to evaluate physician performance for diabetes and other common ambulatory illnesses. The Ambulatory Care Quality Alliance (AQA) has created a "starter set" of prevention measures for ambulatory care (**Table 0-1**). Review this table to see if you are considering these measures in your practice.

A New Approach

A growing number of physicians and other health professionals believe we can overcome these barriers and meet the challenges of quality improvement by employing team-based models of care. In fact, using a team approach has recently been shown to produce measurable improvements in quality of care. A collaborative approach to care may include:

- Using certified diabetes educators and nurse practitioners or physician assistants to partner with physicians to educate patients and help monitor and manage care;

Table 0-1. Ambulatory Care Quality Alliance (AQA) Starter Set—Diabetes

Performance Measure	Definition
Hemoglobin A1C management	Percentage of patients with one or more A1C tests conducted during the measurement year
Hemoglobin A1C management control	Percentage of patients with most recent A1C level >9.0% (poor control)
Blood pressure management	Percentage of patients who had a documented blood pressure in the past year of <140/90 mm Hg
Lipid measurement	Percentage of patients with at least one LDL cholesterol test (or all component tests)
LDL cholesterol level (<130 mg/dL)	Percentage of patients with most recent LDL <100 mg/dL or <130 mg/dL
Eye examination	Percentage of patients who received a retinal or dilated eye examination by an eye care professional (optometrist or ophthalmologist) during the reporting year or during the prior year if patient is at low risk for retinopathy. A patient is considered low risk if all three of the following criteria are met: the patient (1) is not taking insulin; (2) has an A1C <8.0%; and (3) has no evidence of retinopathy in the prior year.

Excerpted from Recommended Starter Set: Clinical Performance Measures for Ambulatory Care. Available at http://www.ahrq.gov/qual/aqastart.htm. Accessed 3 October 2006.

- Providing patients with tools to partner with their care team and help manage their own illness;

- Using innovative systems for improving patient education and follow-up, such as patient registries and group visits for diabetes.

Are you interested in exploring these new approaches? We have developed the *ACP Diabetes Care Guide: A Team-Based Practice Manual and Self-Assessment Guide* to help you succeed. You can use this guide to change your practice and improve the care of your patients with diabetes. Practice change can be tough—it takes patience, persistence, and vision—but its rewards can reinvigorate you and many aspects of medical practice by enabling:

- Improved care and better clinical outcomes for your patients;

- Greater reimbursement under new pay-for-performance quality improvement measures;

- Improved efficiency and job satisfaction for members of the care team;

- Improved patient satisfaction, self-management, and quality of life.

How This Guide Can Help

The *ACP Diabetes Care Guide*, authored by a multidisciplinary team of physicians, nurses, and diabetes educators, presents innovative ways to incorporate collaborative care into a variety of clinical settings. You can use this guide to improve diabetes care in your practice, making copies of selected pages and tools for dissemination and using it as a reference for discussing concepts, devising changes, and overcoming challenges. *The ACP Diabetes Care Guide* includes:

- Specific strategies for office redesign;

- Tips on actively involving patients in treatment decisions and self-management;

- Important topics to discuss with your patients;

- Up-to-date clinical guidance for diabetes care;

- Flow sheets, standing orders worksheets, and other *Tools for Better Practice* for improving your care systems;

- *Tools for Better Health*, which are handouts that you can give patients to support their goal setting and self-management;

- A multiple-choice self-assessment test that will qualify physicians and other members of the health care team for continuing medical education and continuing education credits.

The self-assessment test, presented in an interactive format on the accompanying CD-ROM, follows the American College of Physicians' Medical Knowledge Self-Assessment Program® (MKSAP®) model, which includes detailed explanations for improved understanding. Besides the self-assessment test, the CD-ROM includes downloadable, printable versions of all the tools contained in the Diabetes Care Guide Toolkit at the back of this book. In addition, as part of the ACP Diabetes Initiative, which is a broader program that includes courses and innovative patient education material, the ACP Diabetes Portal (http://diabetes.acponline.org) has been launched. The ACP Diabetes Portal provides links to useful resources and a wide array of information on diabetes for patients, clinicians, and other members of the health care team.

An important component of the program is the Assessment of Chronic Illness Care (ACIC) survey, developed by the Improving Chronic Illness Care program of the MacColl Institute for Healthcare Innovation. This survey, available in an easy-to-use interactive format on the accompanying CD-ROM and on the ACP Diabetes Portal, is the first selection in the Diabetes Care Guide Toolkit. This is a powerful tool for evaluating where your practice is before you begin quality improvement work and for evaluating the effect of the changes you implement. Take some time to complete the survey—you may want to start with just one or two components—to begin the process of thinking about how you could improve your practice's systems for providing chronic illness care.

Trying to change entrenched ways of doing things is never easy—roadblocks can include computer systems that aren't up to the task, personnel who are averse to change, and difficulty in just finding the time to try new things. It's important to start small and prioritize. Make one small change and see how it works before moving on to the next component. After all, as patients with diabetes are repeatedly told, small steps can eventually lead to substantial changes. Small gains lay the foundation for even greater success.

1. Improving the Quality of Care in Your Practice—A Team-Based Approach

Organizing a Diabetes Care Team

How do we improve the care of our patients with diabetes?

Up to 95% of patients with type 2 diabetes receive their care from primary care providers. Studies have found few systematic differences in the quality of care provided to patients with diabetes based solely on the specialty of their provider (generalist vs. specialist). Studies *have* found that high-quality diabetes care requires:

- A systematic and organized approach;

- Effective coordination and collaboration among all available personnel within a practice and with external resources (specialists, diabetes educators)—*a team-based approach*.

To improve diabetes care, we need to develop collaborative partnerships with individual patients and actively involve patients in their own care. As we emphasize throughout this care guide, patients' self-management of their diabetes is an essential precondition for improved outcomes. To ensure that our patients receive the best possible diabetes care, we need to redesign our practices to support effective partnerships between all members of a practice team and patients. Successful implementation of the treatment recommendations outlined in the rest of this care guide depends critically on a well-organized practice environment.

The first step in improving the quality of your practice's diabetes care is to assess how you are currently doing and identify which areas need improvement. The Assessment of Chronic Illness Care (ACIC) Survey was developed by the Improving Chronic Illness Care program for this

purpose. The survey can be found in the *Diabetes Care Guide Toolkit [Assessment of Chronic Illness Care (Diabetes)]*. An interactive version of the survey can be found on the CD-ROM that accompanies this book. Support materials to help you identify and eliminate weaknesses in your approach to diabetes care are also available at the ACP Diabetes Portal (http://diabetes. acponline.org).

Just as important as defining areas in need of improvement is enlisting the support of champions for organizational change. These champions play a crucial role in advocating for improvement and spreading enthusiasm to the rest of the practice.

Ideally, such champions should include a doctor, a nurse, and an administrator. Diffusion and acceptance of recommended changes by all members of an office are vital to success.

What are the steps involved in reorganizing our practice to provide high-quality, team-based diabetes care?

To improve chronic illness care, a health system—whether a primary care practice, a midsized physician network, or a large ambulatory care network—needs to develop a culture that supports improvement and is prepared for change at all levels, beginning with the senior leadership. The Chronic Care Model (www.improvingchronic care.org/change/index.html) outlines the basic elements for improving the care of chronically ill patients and is an excellent resource for enacting practice changes to improve care. A medical practice does not have to immediately implement changes in all the areas mentioned to improve care—practices should start with one key area (for example, developing a registry of all patients with diabetes) and then incrementally build on that. Specific steps in developing a diabetes care team include the following steps:

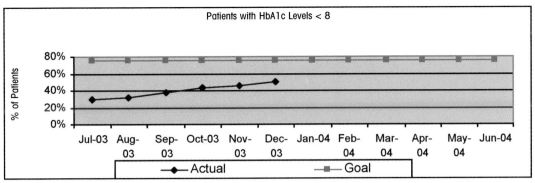

Figure 1-1. **Measuring Progress** This graph monitors improvement in the care of patients with diabetes.

Adapted with permission from Improving Chronic Illness Care: Improving Your Practice Manual, 2005:15. Available at: www.improvingchroniccare.org/ improvement/sequencing/Introduction.htm. Accessed 3 October 2006.

1. **Assign responsibilities.** Determine clear roles and responsibilities for the care of patients with diabetes and other chronic illnesses. Each member of your care team should know exactly who does what and when at the time of a diabetes visit.

2. **Develop a patient registry.** Build a database that helps you identify all patients with diabetes and their key clinical data, and keep your database updated. Such a patient registry provides necessary information to deliver evidence-based diabetes care on a regular, proactive basis. It also helps monitor and report performance.

3. **Track your progress in improving care.** Choose measures to track your improvements. These may be clinical outcomes measures, such as hemoglobin A1C, blood pressure, and LDL cholesterol levels, or process measures, such as completion of routine screening. Create a system of standing orders and reminders to facilitate proactive care. By regularly updating clinical data in your registry, you can monitor the effort you make to reach the goals you have established for each measure. For example, a template available at www. improvingchroniccare.org/improvement/ docs/Diabetes_Reporting_Template.xls lets you plug in the monthly numbers for your diabetes population to generate graphs such as **Figure 1-1**. Other tools that will help you meet your goals are included in Chapter 1 of the *Diabetes Care Guide Toolkit*:

- ⊛ *Standing Orders*
- ⊛ *Diabetes Care Flow Sheet*
- ⊛ *Diabetes History and Self-Management Checklist*
- ⊛ *Diabetes Eye Examination Report*
- ⊛ *Drugs for Primary or Secondary Prevention of Cardiovascular and Kidney Disease Checklist*

Information on available tools to facilitate medical record abstraction is available at: www.takingondiabetes.org/practices/ toolkit.htm. Other useful tools for tracking your progress in improving diabetes care are available at: www.betterdiabetescare. nih.gov/MAINtoolbox.htm.

4. **Implement a system for planned visits for diabetes care.** Be sure your practice has a system for bringing diabetes patients in for regular, planned visits specifically to address diabetes. These can be one-on-one or group visits.

5. **Incorporate diabetes self-management education and support into every visit.** Develop a system to provide self-management education at every visit and ongoing self-management support. Systems need to be put in place to enable patients to set realistic diabetes goals in collaboration with the care team and to follow up regularly to address problems and set new goals. **Table 1-1** provides an example of team care for diabetes. It is also important to establish a

Table 1-1: Team Care of Patients with Diabetes

1. Initial team visit
• Medical history and physical
• Laboratory evaluation
• Risk factor assessment
• Nutritional assessment
• Physical activity assessment
• Psychosocial assessment
• Educational assessment
2. Intervention
• Self-management education and support/referral for diabetes education and medical nutrition therapy
• Collaborative goal setting for metabolic and self-care goals
• Plan for ongoing contact between patient and appropriate team members
• Referral to specialists as necessary
3. Ongoing team care
• Assessment of progress toward goals and self-management
• Identification of barriers to self-care
• Problem solving, including adjustments in therapy and self-care goals
4. Annual planned team visit
• Annual examination for complications assessment
• Reassessment of medical, nutritional, educational, and psychosocial needs
• Revisiting metabolic goals

Adapted with permission from Team Care: Comprehensive Lifetime Management for Diabetes. National Diabetes Education Program. Available at www.ndep.nih.gov/diabetes/pubs/TeamCare.pdf. Accessed 3 October 2006.

system to ensure adequate referral to community and other support programs.

6. **Support the use of evidence-based guidelines.** Clinicians need convenient access to the latest evidence-based guidelines for diabetes care, and these guidelines should be incorporated into daily practice through the use of standing orders and reminders. (The *Standing Orders* and *Diabetes Care Flow Sheet* tools in the *Diabetes Care Guide Toolkit* incorporate current diabetes care guidelines.) Continual educational outreach to clinicians reinforces the use of these standards. You can encourage patient participation by sharing evidence-based guidelines with them. See *Elements of Team-Building in a Clinical Practice*.

Who Does What?— Defining and Delegating Practice Team Roles

From a 2-person office to a 10-person specialty group, a collaborative, well-functioning team is essential for high-quality diabetes care. It is important to define and delegate specific tasks to both clinical and nonclinical staff. Some steps for achieving this outcome are listed below:

1. Review with all team members the guidelines and expectations for care that you have decided to prioritize. Decide which parts of the guidelines may need to be adapted to your local setting. Discuss how the team as a whole can be involved in implementing each process within the guideline.

2. For each guideline, it may be useful to clearly delineate exactly who will carry out each necessary task. **Table 1-2** provides an example of assigning responsibilities for the evidence-based guideline of annual screening for neuropathy with a monofilament sensation test. (*Implementing Clinical Guidelines* in the first chapter of the toolkit provides a blank form you can use to assign specific responsibilities.)

3. To organize planned visits for patients with diabetes, you can use a similar roles grid to identify the logistic and clinical tasks necessary for the preparation and execution of the visit (**Table 1-3**).

4. Clear delineation of roles is especially important for incorporating self-management education and support into routine office visits. For self-management support to be provided in an office-based practice, systems must be established to ensure that this support is incorporated into the flow of the visit. Physicians can serve as important catalysts and reinforcers of diabetes self-management. However, in light of the multiple competing demands of short office visits, physicians cannot be expected to provide the bulk of self-management education support. For

Elements of Team-Building in a Clinical Practice

DEFINE GOALS:

1. Establish an overall organizational mission statement. For example:

- Improve patients' health and outcomes.

- Reduce barriers to access to care.

- Improve practice's financial performance.

- Increase physician and staff satisfaction.

- Improve patient-centered care and patient satisfaction.

2. Establish specific, measurable operational objectives. For example:

- At least 80% of patients with diabetes in a practice will have hemoglobin A1C values lower than 8.0%.

- At least 90% of people calling for a nonurgent appointment will receive an appointment within 1 week.

- Our practice will achieve a targeted level of practice revenue.

- Each team member will achieve an explicitly identified goal for professional development.

- Satisfaction will be evaluated based on appointment keeping, return for follow-up appointments, and achievement of patient-selected self-management goals.

CREATE EFFECTIVE SYSTEMS:

1. Establish clinical systems. For example:

- Implement procedures for providing prescription refills.

- Implement procedures to determine how decisions are made in the practice.

2. Establish administrative systems. For example:

- Create procedures for making patient appointments.

- Create policies for how decisions are made in the medical practice.

CREATE A DIVISION OF LABOR:

1. Define tasks.

2. Assign roles after determining which team members perform which tasks within the clinical and administrative systems of the medical practice.

ENSURE PROPER TRAINING:

1. Provide training for the functions that each team member routinely performs.

2. Initiate cross-training by providing additional expertise needed for team members to substitute for multiple staff members when absences, vacations, or periodic heavy demands affect specific parts of the team.

ENSURE CLEAR LINES OF COMMUNICATION:

1. Establish communication structures. For example:

- Create effective routine communication through paper and electronic information flow.

- Ensure effective minute-to-minute communication through brief verbal interactions among team members.

- Set up team meetings.

2. Establish communication processes. For example:

- Provide feedback.

- Create methods for resolving conflicts.

Adapted with permission from Improving Chronic Illness Care: Improving Your Practice Manual. Available at: www.improvingchroniccare.org/improvement /sequencing/Introduction.htm. Accessed 3 October 2006.

Table 1-2. Example: Assigning Responsibilities for Implementing a Clinical Guideline

Guideline being implemented: _Diabetic Foot Examination_		
Task	**Person Responsible**	**When/How/Why**
Foot sticker placed on front of chart for all patients with diabetes	Front Desk	At check-in/on MD's advice; after a new diagnosis
Determine date of last foot exam	Medical assistant or person taking vitals	Taken from flow sheet in chart. Annual exam unless otherwise noted Flow sheet placed on front of chart
Shoes and socks removed (if due)	Medical assistant or person taking vitals	Date of last exam triggers removal of socks and shoes
Explanation of foot exam (when needed)	Medical assistant or person taking vitals	As shoes and socks are being removed and other vitals being assessed
Monofilament placed on top of chart	Medical assistant or person taking vitals	To make sure right equipment is at hands of provider
Sensate test performed	Trained provider (RN, PA, NP, MD)	Results recorded on flowsheet

Reprinted with permission from Improving Chronic Illness Care: Improving Your Practice Manual. Available at: www.improvingchroniccare.org/improvement/sequencing/Introduction.htm. Accessed 3 October 2006.

example, assistants can mail patients reminders about previously set self-management goals and other information in advance of their visits. Assistants can also arrange for patients to complete self-management forms in the waiting room. Nurses can facilitate efficient examinations, and nurses and diabetes educators can review self-care issues in follow-up discussions with patients. The tools in Chapter 2 of the _ACP Diabetes Care Guide Toolkit_ will help you meet your objectives.

5. Provide patients with information regarding effective community programs and encourage them to participate. Community resources—schools, government programs and agencies, nonprofit groups, and faith-based organizations—can bolster our efforts to keep patients with diabetes or other chronic illnesses supported, involved, and active. Form partnerships with organizations such as churches or senior centers to fill gaps in providing needed services, including exercise programs, food demonstrations, and support activities, such as peer counseling and support groups.

Until new roles are well-integrated into the normal work flow, your team may benefit from 5- to 10-minute team meetings each morning to review the schedule and to identify diabetes patients with visits that day. You should also address team member roles for those visits.

Integrating Self-Management Support into Clinical Practice

There is no substitute for integrating effective self-management education and support into the ongoing medical care provided to diabetes patients. More intensive self-management support, however, is often required. In particular, diabetes patients need intensive initial diabetes self-management education. Such education can be provided most effectively by health professionals—such as diabetes educators and dietitians—who have the knowledge and time to offer patients the skills and support required to carry out the range of tasks required for diabetes self-management. Individual practices must have systems in place to ensure that patients are referred to these more intensive education and support programs.

Table 1-3. Example: Assigning Responsibilities for a Planned Diabetes Office Visit

Task	Person Responsible	When/How/Why
Call patients to schedule planned visit.	Medical assistant	Use diabetes registry to identify patients.Call higher-risk patients with abnormal values first.Make sure all diabetes-related issues can be addressed adequately in visit.
Perform preliminary intake.	Medical assistant	Before visit with trained provider
Remove shoes and socks.	Medical assistant	After vital signs are taken and after patient is in examining room
Perform and record foot examination.	Trained provider (RN, PA, NP, MD)	During physical examination
Update results of prior tests.	Trained provider (RN, PA, NP, MD)	During office visit, using data sheet attached to record
Update list of necessary screening tests.	Trained provider (RN, PA, NP, MD)	At end of office visit, using data sheet attached to record
Discuss self-management goals.	Trained provider (RN, PA, NP, MD)	During office visit
Follow up and record patient's self-management progress.	Nurse	Telephone call approximately 2 weeks after visit, using field in registry to identify patients who need to be called

- All patients with recently diagnosed diabetes should be referred to dietitians for consultations and to a formal diabetes education program.

- Practices should have ties to formal diabetes self-management training programs and diabetes educators who can provide ongoing training and additional support to patients.

- A system should be created in your practice to assess self-management and the need for additional education and support annually.

The following two Web sites have information on diabetes education programs and educators throughout the country: www.diabetes.org/education/edustate2.asp and http://members.aadenet.org/scriptcontent/map.cfm.

How do we make these changes in the context of a busy clinical practice?

Rather than trying to make multiple changes at once, take incremental steps, developing a list of priorities and then testing one new change at a time. The PDSA (Plan-Do-Study-Act) cycle is a widely used method for rapidly testing a change—by planning it, trying it, observing the results, and acting on what is learned (**Figure 1-2**). The key principle behind the PDSA cycle is to test on a small scale and to test quickly (see *The PDSA Cycle in Action*).

Plan—Define your objectives, decide the details of who, what, where, and when, and make predictions about what will happen and why.

Do—Execute the plan on a small scale and see how it works. Document experiences, problems, and surprises that occur during the test cycle.

Study—What have you learned? Evaluate the results and adjust the plan if necessary.

Act—Enact the change if the experiment was a success. Are there are any refinements or modifications needed to the change you have tried? This may lead to additional test cycles, starting the process over again with *plan*.

For more information on using the PDSA cycle for improvements in clinical practice, go to www.ihi.org/IHI/Topics/Improvement/ImprovementMethods/HowToImprove.

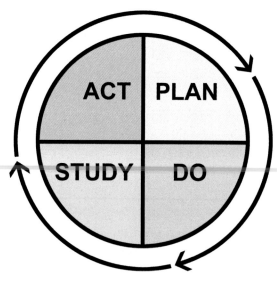

Figure 1-2. **PDSA cycle** The Plan-Do-Study-Act cycle is a widely used method for rapidly testing a change.

Patient Registries

How do we select and use a registry for patients with diabetes?

Organizing patient data is crucial for improving diabetes care. A registry—a disease-specific database of patient information—lets you monitor patient health status and screen for complications, with the ultimate goal of improving intermediate and long-term outcomes. For example, if a registry is in place, all patients whose last hemoglobin A1C value, LDL cholesterol level, or blood pressure was high could be easily identified to ensure that they return to the office for adequate follow-up.

Registries differ from electronic health records (EHRs) in that they manage only selected information relevant to a given condition rather than more comprehensive information about patient problems and history. A registry may be integrated with an EHR or maintained as a separate program that can be used with paper charts in offices without an EHR. There are public domain as well as proprietary registry programs available to use in practice. The CD-ROM that

The PDSA Cycle in Action

If a practice develops a registry of all patients with diabetes, it may then experiment with different strategies for using the registry to identify and contact patients who require follow-up in specific areas. One PDSA cycle might focus on identifying and contacting a limited number of patients—perhaps 20—who have not had a dilated eye examination within the recommended interval. Practice members would develop a plan of who in the office would gather the registry information, who would contact patients, what steps would be taken to refer patients for dilated eye examinations, how information would be documented, and who would follow up to assess whether the patients received the service. During and after the PDSA cycle, the involved staff would identify problems.

accompanies this workbook includes a tutorial for selecting and implementing a registry to improve the care of chronically ill patients, such as those with diabetes.

Patient registries are generally designed to deliver three types of reports:

1. **Patient reports.** Provide patient- or condition-specific information, prompt the user to conduct appropriate assessments, and offer decision support based upon clinical guidelines and patient concerns. Useful for maximizing patient visits.

2. **Registry exception reports.** Identify patients with apparent gaps in care who are overdue for evaluation or are not meeting treatment goals. Useful in developing appropriate outreach strategies for each patient.

3. **Aggregate reports.** Provide aggregate data with regard to desired outcome measures. Useful in gauging progress of care team in meeting treatment goals and improving care.

Computerized databases provide an efficient way to store patient data and enable summaries of care to be printed during the visit. These printed summaries can then be used to collect new data to update the registry, and patient population data can be extracted for a monthly report to track your progress in managing all patients with diabetes. Registries enable you to be better prepared for patient visits and can simplify charting. A computerized registry is ideal, but even a well-designed paper-and-pencil system using index cards can greatly improve care. An example of a card-file registry can be accessed at www.improvingchroniccare. org/tools/criticaltools.html.

Group Visits

How do we incorporate group visits into our practice?

Group visits bring patients who have the same chronic condition and who face similar self-management challenges together with a health care provider or team of providers. Group visits are a highly effective and efficient way to enhance diabetes management and self-management support. They incorporate many of the core components of high-quality chronic disease care, such as:

- Planned, scheduled contact with a care manager or physician

- A targeted focus on improving necessary self-management skills

- Patient support from other patients facing similar self-management challenges

- Use of information systems to support treatment priorities

Many models of group visits lend themselves to a variety of practice settings and outcome goals. For example, models specifically designed to increase self-management support have led to improved physiologic outcomes in diabetes and other chronic conditions, improved self-efficacy and satisfaction, and decreased emergency department use and hospitalizations.

Types of Group Visits

Some examples of effective models follow. These are intended to illustrate various models; you can modify these based on your own practice needs and setting. For a more detailed comparison of these models, go to www.improvingchronic care.org/tools/criticaltools.html.

Cooperative health care clinic: Monthly group meetings (1.5–2 hours) of 15 to 20 patients staffed by a primary care provider, a registered nurse or a diabetes nurse educator, and occasionally by ancillary staff (pharmacist, physical therapist, dietitian). After a 45-minute warm-up and presentation on a selected topic (selected by the provider or by the group), providers circulate and triage patients during a 15-minute break. Fifteen minutes are allotted for questions and answers and 30 minutes for brief one-on-one time with the physician.

Drop-in group medical appointment (DIGMA): The group may meet weekly or monthly. Staffing for the DIGMA consists of the primary care provider, a medical assistant, and a psychologist (some sites use a social worker or a registered nurse). During the 90-minute visit, the assistant checks vital signs and does chart retrieval, and the psychologist conducts warm-up until the provider arrives. Patients are interviewed in a room sequentially, and the provider "huddles" with patients while the psychologist discusses topics with the group. Topics are determined by the medical issues of attendees. The psychologist emphasizes commonalities, self care, and coping skills.

Continuing care clinic (also called *chronic care clinic*): Half-day clinic three or four times per year for a group of eight patients. Group members receive one-on-one time with the primary care provider, pharmacist, and nurse. The group also participates in a self-management–focused group session staffed by a nurse or social worker. Additional information on continuing care clinics is available on the ACP Diabetes Portal (http:// diabetes.acponline.org).

Cluster visits: Two-hour monthly visits that focus on self-management and are led by a diabetes nurse educator, with between-visit proactive phone calling. The group consists of 10 to 18 patients. During a 6-month program, various diabetes team members (podiatrist, pharmacist, nutritionist, etc.) assist. The primary care provider reviews cases.

Chronic disease self-management program: Weekly sessions (six or seven) for 10 to 16 participants. Each 2.5-hour session, which may take place in a clinic or in a community setting (church, senior center), is led by a lay volunteer and focuses on self-management topics. Sessions are supplemented by telephone calls among participants.

Diabetes support groups: Setting, staffing, and schedules vary widely. Groups may be peer led or professionally led; they provide social and/or educational support and may be highly structured or unstructured. Group size ranges from 8 to 20 members.

Can our practice be reimbursed for group visits?

If physicians, midlevel providers, or nurses participate in the group visits, they can be reimbursed in exactly the same way as they would be for individual appointments. Just as in individual appointments, documentation must match the billing code used. Vital signs and other routine data should be charted. Clinicians participating in the visit must create a progress note, and an ICD-9 and CPT code for each patient service must be entered on an encounter form. The following CPT codes are generally used for follow-up appointments conducted as group visits: *99212*, *99213*, *99214*, and (sometimes) *99215*, depending on the level of service rendered. Several excellent resources provide step-by-step guidance in planning and implementing a group visit for your patients with diabetes. One comprehensive guide is "The Group Visit Starter Kit: Improving Chronic Illness Care," which is available free of charge at: www.improvingchronic care.org/improvement/docs/startkit.doc.

Working with Specialists

When should a patient be referred to a specialist?

Achieving adequate glycemic, blood pressure, and lipid control may require complicated therapeutic regimens and approaches for some patients. Maintaining continuous glycemic control without episodes of hypoglycemia, for example, may call for combinations of different kinds of insulin. And many patients with diabetes will require multiple medications to achieve adequate blood pressure control: the mean number of medications in the Hypertension Optimal Treatment (HOT) trial to achieve a target diastolic blood pressure of less than 80 mm Hg was 3.3. When primary care providers cannot achieve adequate control or need additional expertise in treating patients with diabetes, they need to have strong working relations with appropriate subspecialists, such as endocrinologists, cardiologists, and nephrologists. Key elements for this essential collaboration between generalists and specialists in diabetes care include:

- Defining clearly the question/problem area that needs to be addressed when making a referral;

- Providing clear documentation about what changes in management have been recommended and made and following up as necessary on whatever changes were made (For example, if a specialist makes a change in a medication that requires laboratory follow-up, the specialist should make sure that the appropriate tests are ordered and completed and that the results are followed up with the patient.);

- Being open to innovation. In areas where specialist resources are scarce, innovative models have been successful, such as having a specialist provide assistance and additional expertise as part of a diabetes expert care team (e.g., a diabetologist and a nurse–certified diabetes educator) that sees patients jointly with primary care teams.

All patients with diabetes should be monitored routinely for the development of nephropathy, retinopathy, and cardiovascular disease. When these are manifest, referral is appropriate. In particular, primary care physicians may consider referral to an endocrinologist when they are out of their "comfort zone" in terms of therapeutic options or practice resources.

Ophthalmology

The presence of diabetes can damage the blood vessels of the retina and lead to diabetic retinopathy. Patients should be monitored closely for this condition, which can lead to severe vision loss and even blindness. Patients with diabetes are also at increased risk of other ophthalmologic conditions, including cataracts and macular edema. Patients with type 1 diabetes should see an ophthalmologist within 5 years of diagnosis or at puberty and annually thereafter, unless findings warrant closer follow-up. Patients with type 2 diabetes should have a dilated eye exam when they are diagnosed with diabetes and annually thereafter, or more frequently as indicated. Women with diabetes should have an ophthalmologic exam before a planned pregnancy, at least once near the beginning of each trimester, and 6 to 8 weeks postpartum.

Use the *Diabetes Eye Examination Report* in the *Diabetes Care Guide Toolkit* to document updated information on your patient's eye health. You can provide a blank copy of the form that your patient can take to the ophthalmologist, or you can send the form directly to the ophthalmologist. Arrange to get the completed form back so you can keep it in the patient's chart with the other filled-out forms from previous visits to the ophthalmologist.

Endocrinology

Primary care physicians may consider referring patients with type 1 or type 2 diabetes who are using more than one type of insulin to an endocrinologist because titrating prandial and basal insulin requires close follow-up with a diabetes team. All patients who use an insulin pump or who consider switching from a multishot regimen to a pump should be referred to an endocrinologist experienced in pump therapy. Pump management requires significant resources typically not available to a primary care physician.

Nephrology

Patients with a creatinine clearance of less than 60 mL/min, persistent microalbuminuria, proteinuria, hyperkalemia, or difficult-to-control hypertension should be referred to a nephrologist for more aggressive blood pressure monitoring and treatment.

Cardiology

Patients with nonspecific symptoms of fatigue, weakness, shortness of breath, dyspnea on exertion, abdominal pain, or a change in baseline exercise tolerance should undergo electrocardiography. Those with a history of coronary artery disease or who are at very high risk due to multiple additional comorbidities (hypertension, dyslipidemia, microalbuminuria, tobacco use, family history of early coronary artery disease) should have a stress test with imaging. An abnormal electrocardiogram or cardiac stress test should prompt referral to a cardiologist. Patients with dyslipidemia who cannot tolerate statin therapy or those with mixed dyslipidemia may benefit from referral to a lipidologist.

Gastroenterology

If a patient has elevated transaminase levels, particularly in the setting of obesity and diabetes, evaluation by a gastroenterologist should be considered. Patients with diabetes are at risk for nonalcoholic fatty liver disease, which can progress to cirrhosis. Patients with abnormal transaminase levels should have a hepatitis panel performed because there is an association between diabetes and hepatitis C.

Patients with chronic nausea and vomiting or with chronic constipation or constipation alternating with diarrhea should be evaluated for gastroparesis. Those with persistent weight loss and diarrhea should be evaluated for gastroparesis and for celiac sprue, which occurs more often among people with diabetes.

Podiatry

All patients with diabetes can benefit from seeing a podiatrist two or three times per year for routine toenail and skin care. Patients with peripheral neuropathy or peripheral vascular disease are at risk for more advanced foot complications and should see a podiatrist more frequently for more aggressive preventive care.

Psychiatry/Mental Health

There is a high prevalence of diagnosed and undiagnosed depression among patients with diabetes. Although antidepressants often provide effective treatment, patients may also benefit from referral to mental health professionals for cognitive therapy and psychotherapy to help them address the demands of their illness. Providers should develop strong collaborative relations with appropriate mental health professionals to assist in addressing the mental health needs of patients with diabetes.

2. Patient Engagement and Self-Management

The Importance of Self-Management Support

Because diabetes is a largely self-managed illness, diabetes education has long been viewed as an essential component of care.

In the past, the success of patient education and support was judged by patients' ability to be compliant with their treatment program. Education was largely content-driven, and the primary educational strategy was lecturing to patients. The view was that patients would learn what to do and then adapt their lives to fit the recommendations of their health-care professionals.

In recent years, the emphasis has shifted from didactic education to programs that are oriented toward empowerment. An empowerment-based program is patient-centered rather than content-driven and is designed to provide patients with the knowledge and skills they need to make informed choices. In addition, patients are helped to identify and achieve their own goals rather than goals chosen by health-care professionals. This approach acknowledges the expertise of the patient in knowing his or her own values and abilities. Within the empowerment framework, diabetes self-management education is designed to meet the needs identified by the patient or group of patients so that they can become informed, active participants in their own care.

Does outcomes evidence support the value of diabetes self-management education?

The answer to this question is yes. Several meta-analyses have shown that diabetes education is effective for improving metabolic and quality of life outcomes. Research has also shown that whereas no one program is more effective than others, education that incorporates behavioral and affective aspects along with information have better outcomes. The results of the Diabetes Attitudes Wishes & Needs (DAWN) Study showed very clearly that people find their diabetes distressing and difficult, even when they are able to effectively manage the metabolic and other self-care aspects. The respondents in that survey also indicated they wanted more help with these issues from their health-care professionals.

How can I incorporate self-management education and support into my practice?

To be effective, diabetes self-management education and support need to be viewed as part of care and incorporated into each routine visit. Specific strategies for incorporating self-management support into a practice include:

- Using a team of professionals within a practice, system, or community

- Implementing case management

- Using interactive technology to enhance self-management education and support

- Using group or cluster visits

- Using standardized instruments or electronic medical records

These strategies are discussed more fully in Chapter 1, Improving the Quality of Care in Your Practice—A Team-Based Approach.

Patients with Newly Diagnosed Diabetes

Principles of Diabetes Self-Management Education

- Patients may be overwhelmed, frightened, angry, or depressed, and unable to process information. These psychosocial concerns need to be assessed before beginning care and education. A list of possible questions to ask patients to assess these and other concerns is provided in **Table 2-1**.

- Initial education is based on the patient's concerns and questions.

- If barriers to treatment are identified during the assessment of concerns (for example, paying for medications, fear of complications), address these concerns initially.

- Ask more than advise; listen more than lecture.

- Repetition is important.

- Initially, patients need enough information to be safe and to feel safe at home (survival skills).

One model for successful implementation of self-management education and support is Glasgow's "5 As" model (assess, advise, agree, assist, arrange). Because patients with a new diagnosis of diabetes require a great deal of information and support, this model can help the clinician provide and evaluate different components of the interaction. Tips for using the 5 As model with a patient with newly diagnosed diabetes are presented below.

The 5 As for Self-Management in Patients with Newly Diagnosed Diabetes

Assess

The questions you ask in the initial assessment of the patient can inform the ensuing discussion

Table 2-1. Self-Management: Assessment Questions

Approach to the Patient
What language do you prefer to speak? To read?
What is your favorite way to learn (e.g., reading, discussion, videos, computers, group class, individual teaching)?
Where do you get most of your information about health and diabetes?
Do you have difficulty with your hearing or vision, such as reading regular-size print?
How far did you go in school?
Do you have any cultural or religious practices or beliefs that affect how you care for your health and diabetes?
Do you have trouble remembering things?

Emotional State
Have you ever known other people with diabetes? How did it affect them?
How much stress are you experiencing in your life?
Have you felt sad and blue most of the time for the past two weeks? Two months?
What were your thoughts and feelings when you first learned that you had diabetes? What are your thoughts and feelings now?

Support Network
What kind of support do you receive from your family and friends to care for your diabetes?
Who helps you the most to care for your diabetes?
What kind of support do you want and need from your family and friends to care for your diabetes?

Readiness and Strategies for Change
Do you have health problems that you manage other than diabetes? What helps you manage them?
Have you ever lost weight or increased your physical activity? What helped you make those changes? What got in your way?
What are you currently doing to manage your diabetes at home?
On a scale of 1–10, with 10 being the most important, how important is managing diabetes in your life?

Concerns and Areas to Address
Do you ever have difficulty paying for your diabetes supplies or medicines?
What aspects of diabetes are you most interested in learning about?
What is your greatest concern about your diabetes?
What is the hardest thing for you in caring for your diabetes? What is the easiest?
How can I be most helpful to you?

and provide guidance in the areas listed below (see Table 2-1):

- How the patient prefers to receive information

- How the patient is coping with the diagnosis

- What kind of a support network is available

- How ready and able the patient is to implement strategies to manage the disease

- Whether there are barriers to self-management or change

Advise

- Address the patient's fears and concerns before addressing diabetes care and education.

- Address any misconceptions about the disease with respect and cultural sensitivity.

- Teach the patient about his or her role in the care of a chronic disease such as diabetes; discuss your role as well.

- Teach survival skills (e.g., for type 1 diabetes, blood glucose/ketone monitoring, dealing with hypo/hyperglycemia).

- Acknowledge that negative feelings are common and provide reassurance (and information regarding counseling/treatment if appropriate).

- For type 2 diabetes, discuss the "continuum of care" and expected treatment changes over time.

Agree

- Plan a return visit and initial education and self-management support.

- Identify when and whom to call if there is a problem or if additional help is needed.

Assist

- Identify a resource for getting questions answered between visits.

- Identify a resource for addressing barriers and problems if any are identified as concerns during the assessment.

- If the primary intervention is lifestyle changes, use community resources and referrals to assist with the "how"—not just the "what."

Arrange

- Arrange a referral for diabetes self-management education and/or medical nutrition therapy.

What education do patients with newly diagnosed diabetes need in their first visit?

The following "take-home concepts" should be discussed with any patient with a new diagnosis of diabetes:

- Diabetes is serious but manageable.

- Negative feelings—fear, anger, sadness—are common. If the feelings become overwhelming or negatively affect self-care abilities, additional help is available.

- Patients have a role in the self-management of their disease and so need to learn as much as possible about it.

- For type 2 diabetes, there is a continuum of treatment—lifestyle changes, then oral medications, then injectables. The point is to use what works and is needed to manage glucose levels.

In addition, depending on their medical status and treatment plan, patients should be provided with clear (preferably written) instructions regarding the following points:

- What to eat until you see the dietitian

- Blood glucose monitoring

- Acute issues (e.g., hyperglycemia)

- Insulin administration with demonstration and practice

- Hypoglycemia (type 1 diabetes)

- Ketone monitoring (type 1 diabetes)

- When to next contact the office for both routine follow-up and urgent/emergent problems

Ongoing Care of Patients with Previously Diagnosed Diabetes

Because diabetes is a chronic illness, a one-time educational intervention is not adequate. Several meta-analyses have shown that although diabetes education is effective for improving metabolic and quality of life outcomes, traditional knowledge-based programs are not enough to help participants sustain the type of behavioral changes needed for diabetes self-management. Patients need initial diabetes self-management education followed by ongoing diabetes self-management support. The goal is to facilitate patients' self-care and behavior change efforts so that patients become effective daily managers of their diabetes. Ongoing self-management support is important for:

- Helping patients initiate and sustain behavioral changes

- Addressing barriers, concerns, and psychosocial issues

- Screening for depression or anxiety

- Helping patients to continue to learn about diabetes and new treatments as they are needed

Although the initial, comprehensive education may best be done outside the practice setting, the office setting is ideal for ongoing diabetes self-management support, including education and goal-setting to achieve behavior change.

How can I help my patients set self-management goals that they can achieve?

An effective strategy for behavior change is helping patients to establish self-management goals based on their own needs, priorities, and values. The empowerment-based 5-step goal-setting process is an effective strategy for setting goals *with* rather than *for* your patients:

1. What is it about your diabetes care that is causing you the most distress at this time?

2. How do you feel about this issue?

3. What do you want to do about this issue (long-term goal)/how important is it to you to address the problem?

4. What will you do this week (short-term goal)/how confident are you that you can achieve the goal you set?

5. How did it work/what did you learn?

A key to the success of this approach is to encourage patients to think of their short-term goals as a series of behavioral experiments. Experiments provide information and feedback regardless of their success or failure. Therefore, the critical question is not "Were you a success?" but "What did you learn and what will you do or not do differently next time?"

All of these five goal-setting steps may not be possible for many providers within the context of a busy office visit and thus can appropriately be the role of other professional staff members. However, providers can begin each visit by asking patients what concerns they need addressed today and end by asking what they plan to work on between this visit and the next. For strategies to help you support behavior change by your patients, see *Tips for Encouraging Behavior Change.*

The "AADE 7" are the seven critical self-care behaviors identified by the American Association of Diabetes Educators (**Table 2-2**). Worksheets for setting self-management goals provided in the *Diabetes Care Guide Toolkit* include *Setting Your Self-Management Goal* and *Your Self-Management Workbook.*

Principles of Ongoing Diabetes Self-Management Education

- Successful self-management education programs are patient-centered and aim to provide education for informed decision making and behavior change. Goal-setting is a patient-directed, rather than a clinician-directed, activity.

Tips for Encouraging Behavior Change

ONE STEP AT A TIME

Changes are easier to make and more likely to last if patients make them one at a time. A series of small changes can ultimately result in a major change in the patient's self-management and lifestyle.

EASY DOES IT

Focus on changes that your patients believe will work. Changes that are likely to work are ones that your patients feel enthusiastic about and believe strongly that they can carry out.

TAKE SMALL STEPS

For example, if you have patients who drink whole milk and want to try drinking fat-free milk, advise them do it in a series of small changes. They can start by switching from whole milk to 2% milk, then change from 2% to 1%, and then from 1% to skim milk. Making changes like these in steps is a way to help your patients gradually adapt to a larger change.

DON'T GO IT ALONE

Advise your patients to ask for support when they need it. It is hard to make long-lasting lifestyle changes without the support of other people. Often patients think those close to them should know what they want in the way of support without having to be told. If your patients are making changes for their health and want the help of their friends, family, or co-workers, advise them to ask for it. Have them tell the people from whom they want support what they are doing, why it is important, and specifically what they want in the way of help.

PLAY TO WIN

Help your patients identify the behavior changes that will be the most meaningful to them personally. Start with these changes even if as a health-care provider you believe different changes would have a greater positive impact on your patients' health. Patients are more likely to succeed in making changes that are important to them personally than in making changes that the provider thinks are important. After the patient has succeeded in making some personally meaningful changes is when to discuss the changes the provider thinks are important.

Source: Anderson RM, Funnell MM. Tips for Encouraging Behavior Change. Copyright © University of Michigan. Used with permission.

- Programs should be flexible according to the learning styles and needs of the patient. For example, a patient may prefer to read on his or her own rather than attend a class or may prefer one goal-setting tool over another.

- Effective programs are based on the principles of adult education and problem-based learning and integrate psychosocial, behavioral, and clinical content.

- Patients whose providers are positive about education (rather than using it as a punishment) are more likely to participate and benefit.

- Depression is common in diabetes and negatively affects patients' ability to manage their diabetes. Screening for depression and other psychosocial barriers to care is an important component of ongoing support.

Self-management interventions can occur either in group or in individual sessions. Practices with a large number of patients with diabetes can create innovative arrangements with local diabetes self-management education providers in the area. For example, one day a week can be scheduled for bringing in a diabetes educator for

Table 2-2. AADE 7 Key Self-Care Behaviors

Healthy eating
Being active
Monitoring
Taking medication
Problem-solving
Healthy coping
Reducing risks

Developed by the American Association of Diabetes Educators. Adapted with permission from Mulcahy K, Maryniuk M, Peeples M, Peyrot M, Tomky D, Weaver T, et al. Diabetes self-management education core outcomes measures. Diabetes Educ. 2003;29:768–70, 773-84, 787-8 passim.

all patients with diabetes. (For other strategies for using a team-based approach to incorporating diabetes self-management education into your practice, see Chapter 1, Improving the Quality of Care in Your Practice—A Team-Based Approach.) Reimbursement for diabetes self-management education has become more widely available in recent years, particularly for programs recognized by the American Diabetes Association. Practices are also learning strategies for obtaining reimbursement for diabetes self-management support (for example, through group or cluster visits) or using personnel other than the provider.

What topics need to be addressed in ongoing self-management discussions with patients?

It is important to enable patients to take the lead in voicing their concerns and questions about managing their disease. *Identifying Your Concerns* in Chapter 2 of the *Diabetes Care Guide Toolkit* is a questionnaire your patient can fill out before an appointment to help frame the discussion of self-management and clinical issues.

The 5 As model can guide you in providing effective ongoing self-management support.

The 5 As for Ongoing Self-Management Support

Assess

As for newly diagnosed patients, the questions you ask your patiens will inform the ensuing discussion.

- What are your greatest concerns at this time about your diabetes? What is hardest for you in caring for your diabetes right now? What questions do you have today? How can I be most helpful to you? What are your thoughts and feelings about diabetes at this time?

- How well do you think your treatment plan is working to manage your diabetes? What do you think would help to improve the situation?

- Have you ever received diabetes self-management education? What was your experience? Are you interested in receiving diabetes self-management education?

Advise

- Explain that negative feelings (fear, anger, sadness) are common but if the feelings become overwhelming or negatively affect self-care abilities, additional help is available.

- Provide information about new therapies and issues as they arise (e.g., starting insulin).

- Provide specific information about the patient's test results.

- Establish priorities for teaching that are based on patient-identified concerns and treatment.

- Use teachable moments and opportunities during the visit for education (e.g., during monofilament testing, point out areas of the foot for which particular attention is needed).

Table 2-3. American Diabetes Association Content Areas for Diabetes Self-Management Education

Describing the diabetes disease process and treatment options
Incorporating appropriate nutritional management
Incorporating physical activity into lifestyle
Using medications (if applicable) for therapeutic effectiveness
Monitoring blood glucose level and urine ketones (when appropriate), and using the results to improve control
Preventing (through risk-reduction behavior), detecting, and treating chronic complications
Goal setting to promote health, and problem solving for daily living
Integrating psychosocial adjustment into daily life
Promoting pre-conception care, management during pregnancy, and gestational diabetes management (if applicable)

Adapted from Mensing C, Boucher J, Cypress M, Weinger K, Mulcahy K, Barta P, et al. National standards for diabetes self-management education. Task Force to Review and Revise the National Standards for Diabetes Self-Management Education Programs. Diabetes Care. 2000;23:682-9.

Address the diabetes self-management education content areas identified by the ADA (**Table 2-3**) either through a formal program or an informal program. (A curriculum titled *Life with Diabetes: A Series of Teaching Outlines* is available from the ADA at: www.diabetes.org/ for-health-professionals-and-scientists/ recognition/resources.jsp.)

- Content areas need to be addressed in order of patient interest and assessed need.

- Not all patients need all content areas.

- Written materials should reflect the culture and literacy level of the audience.

- Written materials need to be reviewed and discussed with patients.

Additional or more specific content areas that may arise include:

- Psychosocial issues

- How to make behavioral changes

- The meaning of numbers (e.g., blood pressure, A1C)

Sick Day Recommendations

KEY MESSAGES FOR PATIENTS ABOUT SICK DAYS INCLUDE THE FOLLOWING RECOMMENDATIONS:

1. Never omit diabetes medication.

2. Self-monitor blood glucose every 3 to 4 hours and perform ketone testing when two blood glucose readings are greater than 250 mg/dL.

3. Drink 6 to 8 ounces of fluids each hour while awake.

4. Call a health-care provider if vomiting or diarrhea persists more than 8 hours, the ketone value is moderate to large, blood glucose values greater than 250 mg/dL do not decrease with extra insulin, blood glucose values are low, or the appropriate action is unknown.

- Standards of care and annual testing

- Moving from pills to insulin (patient decision making)

- Injection techniques

- Hypoglycemia (type 1 diabetes)

- Strategies for remembering to take medications

- Sick day management (see *Sick Day Recommendations*)

- Foot care

- Sexual health

- Simple meal-planning strategies

- Stress management

- Wearing diabetes identification

- Financial resources

- Resources in the community

Agree

- Schedule a return visit and a plan for diabetes self-management education and support.

- Patients should establish self-selected short-term goals, which are followed up at or between visits using the 5-step goal-setting model.

- Establish target metabolic goals and times when a patient is to contact office staff.

Assist

- Identify a resource for getting questions answered between visits.

- Assist patients to identify barriers/problems and identify strategies to address these problems.

Arrange

- Ongoing support through visits, support groups

- Method for follow-up education or support

3. Screening and Diagnosis of Diabetes

Types of Diabetes

How is diabetes classified?

Patients with any form of diabetes may require insulin treatment at some stage of their disease. The use of insulin, in itself, does not classify the type of diabetes.

Type 1 Diabetes Mellitus

Type 1 diabetes is characterized by a beta cell destructive process that is either autoimmune or idiopathic and may eventually lead to absolute insulin deficiency. Although not widely appreciated, type 1 diabetes can occur at any age. Multiple studies have shown that the clinical onset of type 1 diabetes occurs more frequently in adults than in children and that it is not unusual for patients to present in their 60s, 70s, and 80s.

Presentation of type 1 diabetes is usually acute or subacute. Classic symptoms are:

- Polyuria
- Polydipsia
- Polyphagia
- Weight loss
- Visual disturbance
- Recurrent vaginal or urinary tract infections
- Fatigue and malaise

In older adults, type 1 diabetes may present in a more subacute or chronic manner and may mimic type 2 diabetes. This form of type 1 diabetes is often referred to as *latent autoimmune diabetes of adults* and is characterized by a slower progression of beta cell loss secondary to autoimmune destruction of the islets.

More than 90% of cases of type 1 diabetes are autoimmune in nature, characterized by insulitis and the presence of autoantibodies against components of the beta cell or insulin itself (e.g., anti-insulin antibodies, glutamic acid decarboxylase antibodies, or islet cell–associated antigen antibodies). These antibodies are frequently present years before the clinical onset of diabetes, and patients ultimately become insulinopenic and dependent on insulin therapy for survival. Approximately 20% of those with type 1 diabetes develop other organ-specific autoimmune diseases, such as celiac disease, Graves' disease, hypothyroidism, Addison's disease, pernicious anemia, and vitiligo. For a discussion of less common autoimmune syndromes, see *Type 1 Diabetes—Learning from Uncommon Diseases*.

The diagnosis of type 1 diabetes is not excluded by age or by the presence of obesity, which usually indicates type 2 diabetes. Depending on the population, 5% to 20% of patients categorized as having type 2 diabetes are actually autoantibody positive, which suggests that they have type 1 diabetes.

Early after diagnosis, patients with type 1 diabetes may go through what is termed the *honeymoon period*, during which they require little insulin for weeks, months, or sometimes even years. During this time, some can control blood sugars by diet and physical activity or by using type 2 diabetes oral medications. The reason for the honeymoon period lies in the remarkable degree of reserves the pancreas has for producing insulin; insulin insufficiency may only become apparent in the setting of additional stresses such as infection or trauma. However, as the autoimmune destruction continues, the honeymoon period eventually ends and the patient requires daily insulin.

Type 1 Diabetes—Learning from Uncommon Diseases

Some understanding of the pathogenesis of immune-mediated diabetes has come from the identification of monogenic forms of diabetes associated with multiorgan autoimmune syndromes. In particular, two rare syndromes have been identified.

APS-I syndrome (autoimmune polyendocrine syndrome type 1, also called *autoimmune polyendocrinopathy candidiasis ectodermal dystrophy* or *APECED*) results from mutations of the autoimmune regulator gene (AIRE). AIRE is a transcription factor that is important in the thymic expression of a number of peripheral antigens, including insulin. This expression is important for the central deletion of autoreactive T cells. About 18% of affected patients go on to develop type 1 diabetes.

The IPEX syndrome (immune dysregulation, polyendocrinopathy, enteropathy, X-linked; also called *X-linked polyendocrinopathy, immune dysfunction, and diarrhea syndrome (XPID)*) results from mutations of the foxP3 gene. This gene is important for the development of regulatory T cells responsible for peripheral tolerance. Most affected children manifest neonatal diabetes. These "experiments of nature" have aided investigators in understanding (at least in a preliminary way) the roles of both central and peripheral tolerance in the development of autoimmune diabetes.

Because the honeymoon period occurs so early after diagnosis, some patients may view the normalization of blood glucose readings as a sign that the diagnosis was a mistake or that they do not really have diabetes. The end of this period can be particularly devastating for these patients, who must then adjust again to the reality of the diagnosis. It is important, therefore, to prepare patients for this possibility and assess their emotional response during and after this phase of the disease.

Type 2 Diabetes Mellitus

Type 2 diabetes is characterized by a combination of insulin resistance and a beta-cell secretory defect. The disease may range from predominantly insulin resistance with relative insulin deficiency to a predominantly secretory defect with or without insulin resistance. With time, progressive beta-cell dysfunction can develop, leading to absolute insulin deficiency (see *Understanding Type 2 Diabetes*).

Most patients with type 2 diabetes are obese or at least have abdominal obesity (high waist-to-hip ratio). Presentation may range from an asymptomatic one to the classic symptoms listed above for type 1 diabetes. The presence of ketoacidosis does *not* exclude the diagnosis of type 2 diabetes, particularly in non-white populations.

Approximately 20% of patients with newly diagnosed type 2 diabetes have established chronic microvascular complications of the disease at presentation; an even higher percentage may have coronary artery disease or peripheral vascular disease at presentation. Indeed, in a prospective study of patients with acute coronary syndromes, 57% were found to have impaired glucose tolerance, and 66% of those who met the criteria for diabetes did not have a previous diagnosis or were not treated.

Diabetes of Defined Etiology

A subset of patients with diabetes have a known genetic defect, syndrome, or environmental insult leading to disease. Some of the causes include:

- Genetic defects of beta cell function (e.g., maturity-onset diabetes of the young [MODY]—see below)

Understanding Type 2 Diabetes

In type 2 diabetes, the plasma insulin concentration (both fasting and meal-stimulated) is usually initially increased, although only relative to the severity of insulin resistance. Early in the disease, patients may even develop compensatory islet hypertrophy, but eventually, the plasma insulin concentration is insufficient to maintain normal glucose homeostasis. Frequently, there is a delay or loss of early-phase insulin release in response to oral glucose. With time, progressive beta-cell dysfunction can develop, leading to absolute insulin deficiency.

The obesity often associated with type 2 diabetes may directly contribute to insulin resistance. Adipose tissue may influence insulin action through release of free fatty acids and by secretion of such adipose-derived proinflammatory peptides as TNF-α, IL-6, and TGF-β and by modulation of hormones, including adiponectin, leptin, and resistin.

Numerous in vitro experiments have demonstrated profound insulin resistance in tissues from obese patients with type 2 diabetes; we are starting to understand the tissue and cellular defects leading to this insulin resistance. Type 2 diabetes also appears to involve numerous downstream defects in insulin receptor signaling, including abnormalities in phosphorylation of the insulin receptor substrate family of proteins. Similarly, PI 3-kinase activity in skeletal muscle is reduced, which correlates with a decrease in whole body glucose disposal.

- Genetic defects in insulin action (e.g., leprechaunism)

- Uncommon forms of immune-mediated diabetes (e.g., stiff-man syndrome)

- Other genetic syndromes (e.g., Wolfram's syndrome)

- Diseases of the exocrine pancreas (e.g., pancreatitis)

- Endocrinopathies (e.g., Cushing's syndrome)

- Drug- or chemical-induced causes (e.g., glucocorticoids)

- Infection (e.g., congenital rubella)

Based on the underlying etiology, the presentation and treatment of type 1 and type 2 diabetes may be similar. Some of these forms of diabetes may be reversible with correction of the underlying problem—for example, a growth hormone abnormality or cortisol excess.

An estimated 5% of persons with diabetes in the United States have an autosomal dominant form of the disease known as *MODY*. Presentation is generally before age 25 but can occur at any age. The cause is diminished insulin secretory capacity due to mutations in the gene for glucokinase, the rate-limiting enzyme in the glycolytic pathway (MODY 2), or in genes for transcription factors involved in regulating the insulin gene (MODY 1, 3, 4, 5, and 6).

Gestational Diabetes

Gestational diabetes is defined as diabetes developing or discovered during pregnancy. Associated with an increased risk of perinatal morbidity and mortality, an increased rate of cesarean delivery, and chronic hypertension in the mother, gestational diabetes is usually asymptomatic and is diagnosed through routine screening during pregnancy.

Women with gestational diabetes carry a high risk for type 2 diabetes—nearly 50% develop type 2 diabetes within 5 years after diagnosis of gestational diabetes (see *Gestational Diabetes, Predictor for Subsequent Diabetes*). A small subset of women with gestational diabetes have positive islet cell antibodies, indicating that they have type 1 diabetes.

Gestational Diabetes, Predictor for Subsequent Diabetes

Because insulin binding during pregnancy is unchanged, increases in insulin resistance during pregnancy are believed to be secondary to postreceptor factors. Defects in glucose transport may also play a role, as GLUT4 transporter numbers are reduced in adipose tissue later in pregnancy. In addition to increased insulin resistance, insulin clearance may increase moderately as the placenta actively degrades insulin. Even in women without gestational diabetes, insulin secretion in the third trimester in response to glucose is 1.5 to 2.5 times greater than that seen in the nongravid state and is accompanied by islet cell hyperplasia.

During the latter half of pregnancy, circulating levels of estrogen, progesterone, and prolactin, as well as the placenta-derived factors human chorionic somatomammotropin and placental growth hormone variant, all increase. The combined effect of these and other hormonal changes is to oppose insulin at peripheral and hepatic sites while at the same time increasing insulin secretion. Gestational diabetes may develop, particularly in women with coexisting defects in insulin secretion or utilization. This is likely why women who develop gestational diabetes are at higher risk to subsequently develop type 2 diabetes.

Diagnosing Diabetes

How is diabetes diagnosed?

Diabetes can be diagnosed in one of three ways:

- Symptoms of diabetes (polyuria, polydipsia, unexplained weight loss) and a casual plasma glucose (any time of day, regardless of fasting status) of ≥200 mg/dL;

- Fasting plasma glucose (after 8 hours or longer of fasting) that is ≥126 mg/dL;

- Plasma glucose ≥200 mg/dL 2 hours after ingestion of 75-g oral glucose (2-hour oral glucose tolerance test).

The American Diabetes Association (ADA) criteria for the diagnosis of diabetes recommends that whichever test is used, it must be repeated on another day to confirm the diagnosis. Practically, if a patient does not seem likely to return to the office for a confirmatory blood glucose test, a single positive fasting or random blood glucose level may be used to initiate diabetes education and referral for medical nutrition therapy. Likewise, if the diagnosis of diabetes is uncertain, management should include education about prediabetes and counseling for

exercise and weight loss to prevent or delay the actual onset of diabetes.

What are the differences among the tests used for diagnosing diabetes?

Fasting plasma glucose and the oral glucose tolerance test (OGTT) are the two most commonly used tests for the diagnosis of diabetes.

Fasting Plasma Glucose

Fasting plasma glucose is used commonly in clinical practice because of its ease of use and low cost. It is currently the ADA preferred test for screening and diagnosis. However, data from the Third National Health and Nutrition Examination Survey (NHANES III) indicate that the test loses sensitivity in older populations characterized by a disproportionate prevalence of postchallenge hyperglycemia.

Oral Glucose Tolerance Test

The glucose load used in the OGTT varies depending on the setting.

- Nonpregnant adults: 75-g load

- Screening for gestational diabetes: 50-g load

• Diagnosis of gestational diabetes: 100-g load

OGTT is not recommended by the ADA as a first choice for diagnosing type 2 diabetes. Although this test identifies more people at increased risk of developing macrovascular disease (especially coronary artery disease), it remains poorly reproducible and cumbersome to perform. OGTT should be performed under the following conditions:

• If diabetes is strongly suspected and other test results are equivocal

• When the fasting glucose concentration is in range for impaired fasting glucose (100–125 mg/dL)

Proper preparation is important for the accuracy of the OGTT. A high-carbohydrate (150–200 g) diet should be followed for 3 days prior to testing.

Hemoglobin A1C

Hemoglobin A1C is widely accepted as a measure of glycemia and is used in monitoring patients with diabetes; however, its use as a diagnostic test is controversial. Although not recommended as a diagnostic test, many clinicians use A1C for screening because of its ease of administration. Several studies have found high sensitivity and specificity for the diagnosis of diabetes, but other studies have found sensitivity and specificity to be inadequate. If the A1C value is to be used for screening, usually a value of 5.8 to 6.0 (depending on the laboratory normal range and sensitivity and specificity desired) is used as a cut-off followed by OGTT for diagnosis.

The advantages of hemoglobin A1C as a screening test are that it can be performed at any time of day without special preparations and that it may provide a more accurate reflection of glycemic status because it includes both fasting and postprandial components. Unfortunately, hemoglobin A1C assays are not yet standardized worldwide, and many conditions, such as hemoglobinopathies, can render A1C results unreliable. Because of this, the Expert Committee on the Diagnosis and Classification of Diabetes Mellitus recommends against their use for the diagnosis of diabetes.

• If A1C is used for screening, it should be remembered that results may fluctuate widely when different testing products are used.

• Elderly patients have a higher risk of post-meal hyperglycemia and may have high A1C results with normal fasting glucose levels. OGTT can confirm the diagnosis in these patients.

What is prediabetes?

Patients with glucose levels that are elevated but do not meet the diagnostic criteria for diabetes have prediabetes. The term *prediabetes* was adopted to highlight the significantly higher risk these patients have of progressing to diabetes. Impaired glucose tolerance (IGT) is associated with a 2-fold increase in risk for cardiovascular disease and mortality. Although patients with prediabetes usually have no symptoms of hyperglycemia, it is now recognized that approximately 10% of them may develop microvascular complications of retinopathy, neuropathy, and nephropathy before meeting diagnostic criteria for diabetes.

A patient with prediabetes may have impaired fasting glucose (IFG), based on results of fasting glucose level, or IGT, based on results of a 2-hour OGTT. The diagnosis of diabetes and prediabetes based on interpretation of fasting plasma glucose and 2-hour OGTT results is shown in **Table 3-1**.

What educational issues should I discuss with patients with prediabetes?

Patients who have a high risk of developing diabetes should be educated about the effectiveness of regular physical activity and modest weight loss in slowing the progression to diabetes. More information on counseling patients about nutrition, exercise, and goal-setting strategies can be found in Chapter 2 (Patient Engagement and Self-Management), Chapter 4 (Preventing

Table 3-1. Diagnosis of Diabetes and Prediabetes

Diagnosis	Fasting Plasma Glucose	2-Hour Oral Glucose Tolerance Test
No diabetes	<100 mg/dL	<140 mg/dL
Prediabetes	100–125 mg/dL	140–199 mg/dL
Diabetes	≥126 mg/dL	≥200 mg/dL

Data from Benjamin SM, Valdez R, Geiss LS, Rolka DB, Narayan KM. Estimated number of adults with prediabetes in the US in 2000: opportunities for prevention. Diabetes Care. 2003;26:645-9.

Diabetes), and Chapter 5 (Helping Patients Make Lifestyle Changes).

- Never tell patients that they have "a little bit of diabetes" or "borderline diabetes." Patients need to know that they have prediabetes, which already has an increased risk of mortality, but that they can do specific things to prevent progression to diabetes.

- Discuss the importance of smoking cessation as a strategy for helping to prevent cardiovascular complications (see Chapter 12, Complications of Diabetes).

- Stress that incremental changes are more long-lasting and effective than sudden, drastic changes in eating and exercise behaviors.

- Ask patients to choose a behavioral goal at the end of your discussion; for example: "Will you do anything between now and our next visit to help lower your risk for diabetes?"

- Refer for education and/or medical nutrition therapy. Some, but not all, insurance plans and managed care organizations offer reimbursement for education and medical nutrition counseling for the prevention of diabetes. Being prepared by first clarifying reimbursement with the diabetes educator or common insurance plans in your area will facilitate referral.

What educational issues should I discuss with patients with a new diagnosis of diabetes?

Diabetes education in newly diagnosed patients can relieve the anxiety associated with misconceptions and fears about the disease. Provide patients with resources for learning more about diabetes and referral for diabetes education and medical nutrition therapy. Of particular importance is a discussion about the patient's role in managing his or her own disease. Ongoing counseling and self-management support with a diabetes educator, dietitian, or the patient's primary care team is important for success.

- At the time of diagnosis, patients with diabetes (type 1 or type 2) experience much distress. These patients report feeling shocked, guilty, angry, anxious, depressed, and helpless. It is important to ask patients how they feel about their diagnosis, what their concerns and fears are, what questions they have, and how you can be of help.

- Provide factual but hopeful messages. For example: "Diabetes is a serious disease, but it can be managed. It is important for you to understand that most of the day-to-day care is up to you. It is common to feel overwhelmed, angry, or frustrated at times, but I am going to do all I can to help you, and we are going to work together to make sure you get the information and help that you need."

- Regardless of the age of the person with diabetes, the diagnosis affects the entire family. If possible, talk with the family members and address their fears, concerns, and questions; encourage them to learn all that they can about the disease as well.

Screening for Diabetes

Who should be screened for diabetes?

Screening for diabetes (as opposed to the diagnosis of diabetes) consists of testing asymptomatic persons who may be at increased risk of the disease. Although screening is best when carried out as part of a health-care office visit, community screening may help identify patients who do not have maintenance health care. Screening is performed to identify those with type 2 diabetes and, in pregnant women, gestational diabetes.

Type 2 diabetes has a prodromal stage during which the patient is asymptomatic but has an increased risk of diabetes-related complications. The onset of diabetes in this population is estimated to occur approximately 4 to 7 years before the clinical diagnosis. For this reason, and because a large proportion of patients with type 2 diabetes have complications at the time of diagnosis, the ADA recommends screening for type 2 diabetes in all asymptomatic people 45 years or older (**Table 3-2**). If screening is negative for diabetes, testing should be repeated at 3-year intervals. In persons with additional risk factors for developing diabetes, screening should begin at a younger age and/or should be performed more frequently.

A recent study has shown that higher fasting glucose levels that are still within the normal glycemic range (i.e., below 100 mg/dL) may act as an independent risk factor for type 2 diabetes among young men. These results underline the importance of screening asymptomatic patients for type 2 diabetes and closely monitoring high-risk patients.

The incidence of type 2 diabetes is increasing in children and adolescents. Starting at age 10 years or at the onset of puberty (whichever is earlier), children at high risk of type 2 diabetes (**Table 3-3**) should be screened by fasting plasma glucose level. As with adults, a positive result (fasting glucose values ≥126 mg/dL)

Table 3-2. Criteria for Screening for Type 2 Diabetes in Adults

1. All asymptomatic adults 45 years and older should be screened every 3 years.
2. Adults with a body mass index ≥25 (≥23 for Asian Americans, according to the International Diabetes Federation and World Health Organization) and with any of the following additional risk factors should be screened more frequently and screening should be started at a younger age:
• Sedentary lifestyle
• First-degree relative with diabetes
• Member of an ethnic group with a high prevalence of diabetes (Hispanic, Asian, American Indian, African American, Pacific Islander origin)
• History of gestational diabetes or have delivered a baby weighing more than 9 pounds
• History of impaired glucose tolerance or impaired fasting glucose
• Hypertension
• Dyslipidemia (HDL cholesterol level <35 mg/dL and/or triglyceride levels >250 mg/dL)
• History of vascular disease
• Polycystic ovary syndrome
• Signs of insulin resistance (e.g., acanthosis nigricans)

Adapted from: American Diabetes Association. Standards of medical care in diabetes—2006. Diabetes Care. 2006;29 Suppl 1:S4-42.

should be repeated on another day to confirm the diagnosis of diabetes. Screening should be repeated every 2 years in patients who do not meet the criteria for diabetes.

Type 1 diabetes causes significant symptoms at onset and thus generally does not require screening. In addition, measurement of autoantibodies related to type 1 diabetes is not recommended for screening outside of research studies owing to the lack to knowledge regarding how to interpret and follow up abnormal results.

Gestational Diabetes

Who should be screened for gestational diabetes?

Whether or not a woman should be screened for gestational diabetes depends on her level of risk, which should be determined at the first prenatal visit.

Low risk: Women with *all* of the following features are at low risk of gestational diabetes and do not require screening:

• Age <25 years

Table 3-3. Criteria for Screening for Type 2 Diabetes in Children

1. Obesity as defined by body mass index >85th percentile for age and sex *or* weight >120% of ideal for height
Plus
2. Any two of the following risk factors:
   - Family history of type 2 diabetes in first- or second-degree relative
   - At-risk race/ethnicity (American Indian, African-American, Hispanic, Asian/Pacific Islander)
   - Signs of insulin resistance or conditions associated with insulin resistance (acanthosis nigricans, hypertension, dyslipidemia, polycystic ovary syndrome)

Adapted with permission from: American Diabetes Association. Type 2 diabetes in children and adolescents. Diabetes Care. 2000;23:381-9.

- Normal body weight

- No family history of diabetes

- No personal history of glucose intolerance

- No history of poor obstetrical outcome

- Not a member of an ethnic group with a high prevalence of diabetes (Hispanic, African American, Asian, Native American, Pacific Islander)

High risk: Women with *any one* of the following features are at high risk of gestational diabetes and should be tested as soon as possible and retested (if initial results are negative) at 24 to 48 weeks' gestation:

- High body mass index

- Personal history of gestational diabetes

- Family history of diabetes

- Glycosuria

Average risk: Women at average risk do not meet the criteria for either low risk or high risk. These women do not need to be screened for gestational diabetes until 24 to 48 weeks' gestation.

Protocols for screening for gestational diabetes follow either a one- or two-step approach (**Table 3-4**).

How is gestational diabetes managed?

Women who have gestational diabetes and women with diabetes who are pregnant should

Table 3-4. Protocols for Screening for Gestational Diabetes

One-step approach: Perform 100-g oral glucose tolerance test (OGTT) test directly on all patients who require screening.
Two-step approach: Perform initial screening test with 50-g oral glucose load. In patients with a glucose concentration >140 mg/dL 1 hour after glucose load, perform 100-g OGTT test.
Criteria for diagnosis: The OGTT test is performed in the morning after an overnight fast of 8 to 14 hours. The criteria for diagnosis after 100-g OGTT are as follows:

Fasting	≥105 mg/dL
1 hour after load	≥190 mg/dL
2 hours after load	≥165 mg/dL
3 hours after load	≥145 mg/dL

Two or more of the plasma glucose values must be met or exceeded for a positive diagnosis of gestational diabetes.

Data from: American Diabetes Association. Diagnosis and classification of diabetes mellitus. Diabetes Care. 2006;29 Suppl 1:S43-8.

be followed closely with the help of a diabetes educator, a diabetologist, an obstetrician familiar with diabetes management, a nutritionist, and a social worker to prevent poor outcomes (see Chapter 13). Insulin is the treatment of choice to control blood glucose in pregnant women. Oral hypoglycemic agents, angiotensin-converting enzyme (ACE) inhibitors, angiotensin receptor blockers, and cholesterol-lowering agents should be stopped as soon as possible, and blood pressure medications should be changed to drugs known to be safe during pregnancy. Evaluation and management of complications of diabetes should be performed before or as soon as possible after the onset of pregnancy. Women with a diagnosis of gestational diabetes should be screened for diabetes 6 weeks postpartum and periodically thereafter.

What educational issues should I discuss with women with gestational diabetes?

All women with gestational diabetes should be referred for diabetes self-management education and medical nutrition therapy, which are covered benefits under most insurance plans. Important areas to discuss with patients include:

- The importance of near-normal blood glucose levels to prevent complications to the baby

- Meal planning to manage blood glucose levels, not to lose weight

- Blood glucose monitoring and how to use the results

- Therapies: lifestyle, then insulin—no oral drugs during pregnancy (Most women are able to stop insulin postpartum because diabetes goes away; in some women, however, the diabetes does not resolve.)

- Increased risk for type 2 diabetes in the future (Patients should be screened periodically for type 2 diabetes and for gestational diabetes early in subsequent pregnancies.)

- Postpartum preventive strategies, such as exercise and returning to prepregnancy weight

- Pre-conception counseling if type 2 diabetes continues

4. Preventing Diabetes

Lifestyle Measures

Can lifestyle changes like losing weight and exercising really help prevent diabetes in at-risk persons?

The answer to this question is yes. Several randomized controlled trials have confirmed the importance of weight loss, increased physical activity, and a high-fiber diet low in calories and fat in slowing the progression of prediabetes (impaired glucose tolerance [IGT] or impaired fasting glucose) to overt diabetes. Health care professionals can play an important role in promoting these lifestyle changes.

At all ages, the risk of type 2 diabetes increases with increasing body weight. The incidence of type 2 diabetes is highest in persons with upper body or abdominal obesity (a waist-to-hip circumference ratio >0.95 in men and >0.85 in women). In addition, numerous prospective studies have found an association between increased physical activity and a lower incidence of type 2 diabetes.

• The Diabetes Prevention Program Research Group found that at 3 years' follow-up, a 6.8-kg (15-lb) weight loss reduced the incidence of diabetes. In this study, diet and exercise that achieved a 5% to 7% weight loss among overweight adults with IGT reduced diabetes incidence by 58%. Participants in this group exercised at moderate intensity, usually by walking an average of 30 minutes a day 5 days a week, and lowered their intake of fat and calories.

• The Finnish Diabetes Prevention Study found that a weight loss of approximately 3.6 kg (8 lb) was associated with a significantly lower incidence of diabetes. A strong correlation was found between a decreased incidence of diabetes and success in losing weight (goal of 5% weight reduction), reducing fat intake (goal of <30% of calories), reducing saturated fat intake (goal of <10% of calories), increasing fiber intake (goal of ≥15 g/1000 calories), or exercising (goal of >150 min/week).

• In a study of more than 42,000 male health professionals, men who ate a diet high in vegetables, fruit, fish, poultry, and whole grains had a modest reduction in risk of diabetes compared with men who ate more red and processed meat, high-fat dairy products, sweets, and desserts. Similarly, a prospective study of 69,554 women age 38 to 63 years found higher rates of diabetes incidence among women who ate more red and processed meats, sweets and desserts, French fries, and refined grains than women who ate more fruits, vegetables, legumes, fish, poultry, and whole grains.

Health-care providers play a crucial role both in alerting patients if their weight puts them in a high-risk category for diabetes and other cardiovascular diseases and in helping them develop a weight loss strategy. Modest weight loss (5%–10% of body weight) and modest physical activity (30 minutes daily) are the recommended goals. For guidance in helping your patients lose weight and incorporate more exercise into their lives, see Chapter 5 (Helping Patients Make Lifestyle Changes) and Chapter 9 (Obesity).

Pharmacologic Approaches to Preventing Diabetes

Have any drugs been shown to prevent diabetes?

Although several studies have examined the use of medications to delay progression to diabetes, pharmacologic agents are not currently recommended for this purpose. The greater benefit of weight loss and physical activity strongly suggests that lifestyle modification should be the first choice to prevent or delay diabetes.

• In the Diabetes Prevention Program study, metformin delayed the development of type 2 diabetes by 3 years (versus 11 years in the diet plus exercise group) and reduced the absolute incidence of diabetes by 8% (versus 20% in the lifestyle modification group). Thus, whereas metformin is an effective prevention strategy, it is not as cost-effective as lifestyle modification without medication. Metformin was nearly ineffective in adults who were older (>60 years) or less overweight (body mass index [BMI] <30). It was as effective as lifestyle modification in adults aged 24 to 44 years or with a BMI ≥35.

• Troglitazone (no longer available because of liver toxicity) reduced the risk of progression from gestational diabetes to diabetes by 56% in the Troglitazone in Prevention of Diabetes (TRIPOD) study.

• In the Study to Prevent Non–Insulin-Dependent Diabetes Mellitus (STOP-NIDDM), the alpha-glucosidase inhibitor acarbose reduced the risk of progression to diabetes by 36% among adults with IGT.

• Eight of ten studies to date have shown that treatment with inhibitors of the rennin-angiotensin aldosterone system in populations at high risk for cardiovascular disease was associated with a significant reduction in subsequent development of diabetes.

There are currently major trials in progress examining the effects of rosiglitazone/ramipril (the Diabetes Reduction Approaches with Ramipril and Rosiglitazone Medications, or DREAM, study), nateglinide/valsartan (the NAVIGATOR study), and pioglitazone (the ACT NOW study) on the development of diabetes in adults with IGT.

5. Helping Patients Make Lifestyle Changes

Medical Nutrition Therapy

The goals of medical nutrition therapy in diabetes are to prevent and treat the chronic complications of diabetes by attaining and maintaining optimal metabolic outcomes, including blood glucose and hemoglobin A1C levels, LDL and HDL cholesterol and triglyceride levels, blood pressure, and body weight. All patients should be referred to a registered dietitian, preferably one with experience in diabetes, for medical nutrition therapy, particularly when lifestyle modification is the primary method of treatment. Reimbursement for these services has improved greatly in recent years for patients with diabetes.

There is no such thing as a "diabetes diet." Meal planning approaches vary based on the type of diabetes, meal-planning goals, and the treatment plan. Plans need to be developed in collaboration with patients based on their usual eating habits, preferred foods, cultural and religious practices and beliefs, metabolic targets, and self-selected goals. Most patients with type 1 diabetes employ advanced carbohydrate counting by using insulin ratios to manage glucose levels. For those with type 2 diabetes, meal planning approaches range from the very simple (such as the plate method) to the more complex (carbohydrate counting). Meal planning is only one method for managing type 2 diabetes, however. Regardless of the reason, patients for whom this form of therapy is ineffective need to progress to the next level of treatment. Therapies for weight loss are discussed more fully in Chapter 9 (Obesity).

What are some examples of meal planning methods for diabetes?

The Plate Method

A simple strategy for nutrition and meal planning for patients with type 2 diabetes that can result in improved metabolic outcomes and weight loss is the plate method. This is a concrete visual tool to estimate portions and the percentage of particular foods. The plate method can be implemented immediately on diagnosis and before the patient sees a dietitian. The most widely used version divides the plate into fourths—one fourth carbohydrates, one fourth proteins and healthy fats, and two fourths (one half) nonstarchy vegetables. A variation of the plate method is to divide the plate into thirds: one third carbohydrates, one third proteins and healthy fats, and one third nonstarchy vegetables. The goal with either version is to eat the same amount of carbohydrates each day in consistent and reasonable proportions. The plate method is an easy approach for patients to use at potlucks, restaurants, and other settings where it may be hard to count carbohydrates. See *Rate Your Plate* in the Diabetes Care Guide Toolkit for a handout that you can provide your patients.

Healthy Food Choices

This meal planning approach encourages people to eat a variety of foods from various categories (meat/fish, dairy, grains, fruits/vegetables, fats, sweets/snacks). The number of daily servings from each group is developed in collaboration with a dietitian. The checklist *Eating Right* is available in the Toolkit to help patients plan to make healthy food choices.

Basic Carbohydrate Counting

Basic carbohydrate counting helps patients get started with the carbohydrate counting system. Carbohydrate foods are identified as starches, fruit, milk, and desserts. The focus is consistency in the timing, type, and amount of carbohydrate-containing foods eaten. Portion size and label reading are fundamental to understanding how to count carbohydrates. Carbohydrates are measured in grams and may be referred to in grams or in servings (1 carbohydrate serving = 15 g of carbohydrate). Insulin adjustment based on basic carbohydrate counting is discussed in Chapter 8 (Insulins and New Injectables).

Advanced Carbohydrate Counting

Advanced carbohydrate counting is often preferred by patients using multiple daily injections or insulin pumps. This approach gives them greater flexibility in both food choices and timing. Patients who are most successful using this approach check their blood glucose at least four times daily and make multiple daily self-management decisions based on their blood glucose levels, food intake, and activity.

The goal of advanced carbohydrate counting is to titrate the insulin dosage to the predicted effect carbohydrates in a meal will have on blood glucose. Referral to a registered dietitian and/or a certified diabetes educator who can work closely with the patient to determine the insulin-to-carbohydrate ratio is recommended. Advanced carbohydrate counting is also discussed in Chapter 8 (Insulins and New Injectables).

Helping Patients Succeed with Meal Planning

What are some guidelines I can give patients regarding meal planning?

Blood glucose levels are directly affected by three factors:

1. Timing:

   - Eat at least three meals or snacks spaced throughout the day.

   - Eat each meal and snack at about the same time each day.

   - Do not skip meals.

2. Portion size:

   - Eat about the same amount at each meal each day.

   - Pay attention to portion sizes.

3. Food composition:

   - Carbohydrates are the main contributor to blood glucose.

   - The total amount of carbohydrate eaten is a strong predictor of glycemic response; monitoring total grams of carbohydrate is, therefore, a key strategy for glycemic control.

   - Using the glycemic index may benefit meal planning over the use of carbohydrate counting alone; however, it does increase the complexity of meal planning for patients, and the results of studies in this area are mixed.

   - Low-carbohydrate diets are not recommended in diabetes. The recommended range of carbohydrate is 45%–65% of total calories. If the patient wishes to lose weight, this percentage may be lower. (See Table 9-3 for specific recommendations.)

   - Alcohol in moderation is acceptable (total of two drinks or less daily for men and one drink or less daily for women).

   - Simple sugar is not forbidden for people with diabetes.

   - The goal is not to follow a diet; the goal is to manage blood glucose, blood pressure, and lipids by whatever means are necessary.

What should I ask my patients at each visit to assess their meal planning?

Some questions to ask patients with diabetes at each visit when assessing their meal-planning activities include:

- How well do you think your meal plan is working to manage your diabetes?

- What helps you use your meal plan? What gets in your way?

- Have you had difficulty using your meal plan? What specific problems have you encountered? What have you tried to solve this problem? What other options do you think might be effective?

- Do you have any questions about your meal plan?

- How can I help most?

What can I say to patients to help them stay more faithful to their meal plan?

Many patients have difficulty sticking to their meal plans. Some suggestions that may help include:

- Create a plan with a dietitian that takes into account your goals, eating habits, likes and dislikes, family, culture, and personally important foods.

- Set realistic goals for each week and reward yourself when you reach them. Goals that focus on eating habits rather than outcomes are more effective—for example, eating a sandwich and an apple for lunch three days this week instead of two sandwiches (versus losing a specified number of pounds). Goal-setting worksheets for patients are provided in chapter 2 of the toolkit (*Setting Your Self-Management Goal; Your Self-Management Workbook*).

- Eating healthy is not a "diet" but a different way to think about food.

- Let your family and friends know how they can be most helpful to you.

- Decide ahead of time how you will handle special events and holidays. Choosing not to use your meal plan is not "cheating." It is making a decision you have both the right and responsibility to make.

Physical Activity

Physical activity generally lowers blood glucose levels for people with either type 1 or type 2 diabetes. In type 2 diabetes, exercise also decreases insulin resistance and may decrease glucose output by the liver. Physical activity also helps people better manage stress by releasing endorphins, which counteract the effects of stress hormones.

The best forms of exercise are those that the patient enjoys, selects, and will sustain. Recommendations are based on the patient's goals, overall health and level of fitness, the presence of complications, and the treatment plan. The American Diabetes Association recommends at least 150 minutes per week of moderate-intensity aerobic physical activity (50%–70% of maximum heart rate) or at least 90 minutes per week of vigorous aerobic exercise (>70% of maximum heart rate). The physical activity should be distributed over at least 3 days per week and should include no more than 2 consecutive days without physical activity. Cardiac stress testing is discussed in Chapter 12 (Complications of Diabetes).

What strategies can I suggest to my patients seeking to exercise more?

Lifetime Physical Activity Model

This approach is appropriate for patients who have been sedentary or who have a negative

---

view of exercise. The goal is to develop a more active lifestyle by accumulating at least 30 minutes of moderate-intensity physical activities throughout the day on most days of the week. Moderate-intensity activities include walking, doing housework, dancing, raking leaves, climbing stairs, and similar tasks. The Centers for Disease Control and Prevention's website "Physical Activity for Everyone" reviews the Lifetime Physical Activity Model recommendations for clinicians and members of the general public (www.cdc.gov/nccdphp/dnpa/physical/index.htm). *Practical Exercise* in Chapter 5 of the Diabetes Care Guide Toolkit can help your patients discover ways to step up their activity level.

10,000 Steps

The goal of this approach is to encourage your patient to build up to walking 10,000 steps in a day, using a pedometer to keep track. Based on a reasonably active person walking 4,000 to 6,000 steps during a day's normal activities, a 10,000-step goal works out to an additional 4,000 to 6,000 steps (2-3 miles) daily, or the equivalent of a 30-minute (or longer) brisk walk. Thus, this approach is another way to accumulate 30 minutes of moderate-intensity activity daily.

The use of a pedometer serves as both a monitor and a motivator for many who use this approach. Encourage your patient to make simple lifestyle choices, such as taking the stairs instead of the elevator, or parking farther away from the store. These alternatives can add valuable extra steps to the daily total. Many web sites are available for consumers interested in the 10,000 Steps Program. A week-by-week approach that emphasizes gradually increasing steps is available at www.walkinginfo.org. A printable log for recording progress can be found at http://www.walkinginfo.org/hf/features/10kday/10kday.htm#10k.

Planned Aerobic Exercise Programs

Another approach is to encourage your patient to engage in 20 minutes or more (in a session) of vigorous-intensity activity 3 or more days per week. Aerobic exercise programs should include 5 to 10 minutes of warm-up activity and 12 to 20 minutes of exercise in which the patient reaches at least 60% of the target heart rate. (See *Calculating Target Heart Rate*.) A cool-down period of 5 to 10 minutes should follow this exercise.

For maximum benefit, aerobic activity sessions need to occur at least three times per week. Aerobic exercise programs tailored to people of all ages and abilities are widely available, at community centers and fitness clubs as well as on television and video. To provide patients with personalized guidelines for the aerobic exercise they have chosen, use *Your Aerobic Exercise Plan* in Chapter 5 of the toolkit.

Anaerobic Exercise Programs

Resistance exercise consists of activities that use muscular strength to move a weight or work against a resistive load. Examples include weight lifting and exercises using weight machines. Resistance training improves insulin sensitivity and lowers blood glucose levels. People with type 2 diabetes who have no contraindications are urged to perform resistance exercise three times a week, targeting all major muscle groups. They should progress to three sets of 8–10 repetitions at a weight that they can't lift more than 8–10 times.

Resistance training may be contraindicated for patients with some complications and health problems (e.g., retinopathy). The Centers for Disease Control and Prevention's program "Growing Stronger" (http://www.cdc.gov/nccdphp/dnpa/physical/growing_stronger/index.htm) guides resistance training for older

Calculating Target Heart Rate

Target heart rate is based on age. To calculate a patient's target heart rate:

1. Subtract the patient's age from 220. This is the maximum heart rate.

2. The target heart rate for moderate-intensity exercise is generally between 50% and 70% of the maximum heart rate. Multiply the maximum heart rate by 0.5 and 0.7 to determine 50% and 70% of the heart rate.

As an alternative to calculating target heart rate, intensity can be determined by the patient's perceived level of exertion. Using this guide, the participant involved in light to moderate activity should still be able to talk in short sentences.

A target heart rate calculator is available on the accompanying CD-ROM and at the ACP Diabetes Portal at http://diabetes.acponline.org.

adults that may also be appropriate for adults with chronic health conditions such as diabetes.

Helping Patients Succeed with Exercise Plans

What are some guidelines I can give patients to help them exercise safely?

- Choose the correct shoes for the activity and make sure that they fit well. Checking the feet after exercise helps to prevent injuries and find problems, such as blisters, cuts, or other injuries that can quickly become more serious.

- Wear or carry diabetes identification, personal identification, treatment for hypoglycemia (such as glucose tablets or sugar packets), and a cell phone (or change for a telephone) when you exercise, especially if you exercise alone.

- Exercise 1 to 3 hours after a meal. Avoid exercising when your insulin is peaking.

- Symptoms of hypoglycemia can be hard to recognize when they occur during exercise because they may be mistaken for overexertion. If you are unsure, stop exercising and check your blood glucose level and/or treat the hypoglycemia.

- Monitor your blood glucose before, during, and after exercise. If your blood glucose is less than 100 mg/dL and you take insulin or an insulin secretagogue, eat 15 to 30 grams of a carbohydrate and check your blood glucose again. Do not exercise until your glucose level is over 100 mg/dL.

- If you have type 1 diabetes and your blood glucose is 250 mg/dL or higher, test your urine for ketones. Do not exercise if you have ketones in your urine. Your blood glucose can go even higher.

How should I tell my patients to manage hypoglycemia during exercise?

Some tips to share with patients about possible hypoglycemia during exercise include:

- Hypoglycemia can occur during, immediately after, and up to 12 to 48 hours after vigorous exercise. Hypoglycemia is rare, however, among patients with type 2 diabetes who are not taking insulin or an insulin secretagogue.

- Engaging in physical activity that is unusual may lead to hypoglycemia: for example, raking leaves, shoveling snow, doing heavy cleaning.

- People with type 1 diabetes may need to eat an exercise snack or decrease their insulin dosage for vigorous exercise.

- Additional carbohydrates may be needed during and after vigorous exercise that lasts for a long period of time.

What should I ask my patients at each visit to assess how they are doing with regard to physical activity?

Some questions to ask patients to assess their success in incorporating more physical activity in their lives include:

- How well do you think your exercise plan is working to manage your diabetes?

- About how often do you exercise each week? If you are not exercising, are you interested in starting to exercise?

- What helps you exercise? What gets in your way?

- Do you have difficulty with your exercise program? What specific problems have you encountered? What have you tried to solve this problem? What other options do you think might be effective?

- Do you have any questions about your exercise program?

- How can I help most?

Can I provide tips to help patients stay more faithful to their exercise plans?

The following tips can be shared with patients to help them stick to their exercise plans:

- Choose an activity that is enjoyable and plan alternatives for inclement weather or other situations (such as frequent travel).

- Set realistic goals for each week and reward yourself when you reach them. For example, walk 15 minutes after dinner 4 days this week.

- Exercise with a partner.

- Schedule exercise on your day planner or calendar just like other events.

- Let your family and friends know how they can be most helpful to you.

6. Monitoring Glycemic Control

Many factors affect the ability of patients to achieve and maintain near-normal blood glucose levels. Collaboratively developed glycemic goals should take into consideration the patient's age, comorbidities, physical limitations, lifestyle, occupation, support system, and financial resources. The patient's ability to recognize and appropriately treat hypoglycemia should be considered as well.

Self-Monitoring of Blood Glucose

Self-monitoring of blood glucose is the most effective way to assess and manage glycemic control in the short term. Such monitoring provides immediate feedback about the impact that food, medication, stress, and activity have on glycemic control. For a checklist that can help your patients monitor their blood glucose regularly, see *Monitoring Your Blood Sugar* in Chapter 6 of the *Diabetes Care Guide Toolkit*.

How often should I recommend that my patients check their blood glucose?

The American Diabetes Association (ADA) recommends that persons with type 1 diabetes self-monitor their glucose at least 3 times daily. Patients with type 1 diabetes who use basal-bolus insulin regimens should self-monitor their blood glucose at least four times daily (e.g., before meals and at bedtime) and use the data they gather to adjust insulin dosages on a meal-by-meal, day-to-day basis. Regardless of treatment regimen, patients with type 2 diabetes need to have a blood glucose meter and know how to use it. Self-monitoring of blood glucose should be done frequently enough to provide feedback about progress toward goals and to help patients recognize when glycemic control

is deteriorating, such as during times of illness or stress.

- There is no consensus regarding the frequency of self-monitoring in patients who are not taking insulin.

- Patients with type 2 diabetes who use insulin, insulin secretagogues (sulfonylureas, meglitinides), or one of the new injectable drugs (exenatide or pramlintide) are at risk for hypoglycemia and may need to monitor more frequently (up to four times daily and/or when symptomatic) compared with those using lifestyle modifications, either alone or in combination with nonsecretagogue oral agents.

- Patients with either type 1 or type 2 diabetes may need to monitor their blood glucose more frequently when there are changes in insulin or medication dosages, activity, or meals, or during illness or stressful events.

Using the Results of Blood Glucose Monitoring

Blood glucose monitoring alone, no matter how frequent, will not lead to improved glycemic control. Improvement in glycemia is rarely achieved unless patients have been shown how to identify glycemic trends and patterns and how to make appropriate adjustments, either independently or with the assistance of a member of the healthcare team. It is important that patients understand their role in analyzing self-monitoring blood glucose records regularly (daily or weekly) to identify trends indicating that medication or lifestyle adjustments may be needed.

What are the goals for fasting and pre- and postprandial blood glucose levels?

The ADA recommends a goal of 90 to 130 mg/dL for preprandial blood glucose levels in adults with diabetes and less than 180 mg/dL for peak postprandial glucose levels. Similarly, the American Association of Clinical Endocrinologists (AACE) recommends that adults aim for a preprandial blood glucose goal of ≤110 mg/dL and a postprandial goal of ≤140 mg/dL.

Establishing *personal* blood glucose targets in collaboration with patients is critically important, however. These personal targets may be the same as those recommended by the ADA or AACE, or they can be modified based on the patient's ability or willingness to achieve this level of glycemic control or on clinical factors, such as the ability to detect hypoglycemia. In patients whose blood glucose and hemoglobin A1C levels are significantly above the recommended values, it is often more effective to set intermediate decrements in blood glucose and A1C targets. Hitting these intermediate targets will then promote a sense of accomplishment and self-efficacy.

The Role of Postprandial Blood Glucose Monitoring

Epidemiologic studies and preliminary intervention studies have demonstrated that postprandial hyperglycemia is an independent risk factor for cardiovascular disease in patients with type 2 diabetes. Because treatment modalities can now target postprandial blood glucose excursions, assessing how well postprandial blood glucose levels are controlled is important for determining when treatment adjustments are needed. Generally, measuring blood glucose levels 2 hours after a meal approximates the peak postprandial blood glucose concentration in patients with diabetes. It is important to measure postprandial blood glucose levels under the following circumstances:

- If hemoglobin A1C is elevated but fasting glucose levels are within the target range

- To determine the adequacy of the pre-meal insulin dosage when using basal-bolus insulin therapy

- If the patient is using an oral agent that targets postprandial glucose excursions, such as repaglinide (Prandin) and nateglinide (Starlix)

- If the patient is counting carbohydrates

- If the patient is making lifestyle modifications (diet and exercise) to achieve optimal blood glucose control

Blood Glucose Pattern Management

Pattern management is a systematic method of analyzing self-monitoring blood glucose data to make appropriate adjustments in the treatment plan. Ideally, all patients with diabetes should learn how to use pattern management to prevent extended periods of hyperglycemia.

Patients use pattern management to assess the effectiveness of their treatment regimen and to make treatment modifications, either independently or with the help of a health-care provider, to bring blood glucose levels back into a predetermined target range. Pattern management enables patients with both type 1 and type 2 diabetes to assume more responsibility for their diabetes management and often leads to improved glycemic control by limiting the magnitude and duration of out-of-target blood glucose levels.

For patients with type 1 diabetes and for insulin-treated patients with type 2 diabetes, pattern management provides the data necessary to make self-directed adjustments in insulin dosages, carbohydrate intake, and/or activity. Pattern management is also useful for patients with type 2 diabetes who are not taking insulin but who are using lifestyle modification, oral agents, or exenatide to manage their diabetes. Pattern management helps these patients recognize when their current treatment is ineffective. Relying on pre-established guidelines, patients can use pattern management to understand when to seek advice from their health-care providers.

Pattern management requires patients (or their health-care providers) to:

- Know their individualized blood glucose target range

- Learn how to review blood glucose records regularly (daily or weekly) to identify any pattern of hypo- or hyperglycemia (usually defined as three or more self-monitoring blood glucose values outside the target range)

- Understand which components of the treatment regimen are responsible for the pattern

- Make adjustments, either independently or with the assistance of a health-care provider, to the treatment regimen that address the identified pattern

Blood glucose patterns are affected by many factors:

- Fasting blood glucose concentrations are influenced by medication or basal insulin dosage, the size of an evening meal or snack, and the amount of physical activity during the previous 24 hours.

- The dawn phenomenon, defined as an increase in blood glucose levels during the early morning hours (4 AM–8 AM), can have a pronounced effect on fasting blood glucose concentrations. It is thought to be related to increased levels of growth hormone at this time. The dawn phenomenon is seen more often in patients with type 1 diabetes than in patients with type 2 diabetes. Less commonly, fasting hyperglycemia is attributed to antecedent, nocturnal hypoglycemia (the Somogyi effect or *rebound hyperglycemia*).

- Postprandial blood glucose concentrations are influenced by the dosage of the pre-meal medication (either an oral secretagogue or rapid-acting insulin), the carbohydrate content of the meal, the preprandial blood glucose concentration, and physical activity.

Methods of pattern management for patients on insulin are described in more detail in Chapter 8 (Insulins and New Injectables). Patients using oral medications and those who are unable or unwilling to make insulin adjustments based on self-monitoring blood glucose results need instructions on how frequently to contact their providers. This is necessary to routinely review their blood glucose records. These patients also may need specific guidelines about out-of-target readings. Patients initiating any changes in their regimen need similar guidelines.

What are some of the barriers that prevent patients from monitoring their glycemic control as recommended?

Financial

- Most test strips cost about 75-80 cents each.

- Some insurance companies limit the number of test strips permitted each month.

Fear

- Monitoring is a reminder of the diagnosis and the risk for complications.

- The patient views the results as a judgment of his or her self-management efforts rather than as data.

- The patient fears criticism from his or her health-care provider. (It is very common for patients to want their provider to think well of them.)

- The patient fears that the provider will not provide the same quality of care if the patient is not doing his or her part.

- Elevated results may mean that the diabetes is worse or that insulin is needed.

Discomfort associated with fingersticks

- Some patients experience more discomfort than others.

- Alternate-site testing can often eliminate or reduce discomfort.

Inconvenience

- Patients who are unwilling or unable to self-monitor blood glucose in public may not be able to find a suitable place to do the monitoring.

- Carrying the needed supplies can be cumbersome.

- Self-monitoring blood glucose interrupts activities of daily life.

Not seen as important

- The patient has not been adequately informed about the utility and importance of self-monitoring blood glucose.

- The patient has not been taught how to use the information from the results.

- The patient views the monitoring as unimportant because the health-care provider does not ask for his or her self-monitoring blood glucose records, does not review them when the patient brings them to an appointment, or uses them to criticize the patient's efforts.

- The patient sees no changes in self-monitoring blood glucose results or hemoglobin A1C values despite making lifestyle modifications and monitoring as often as recommended.

What should I include in my discussions with patients about blood glucose monitoring?

There are several things you can do when discussing self-monitoring of blood glucose with patients:

- Stress that the purpose of monitoring is for the patient to use results for daily decision making. Therefore, results should be recorded accurately (see *When Patients' Blood Glucose Logbooks Are Inaccurate*). The results also provide information for providers, but the primary user of the daily information is the patient.

- Ask patients what they think the results mean (rather than just telling them).

- Remind patients that self-monitoring blood glucose results are not used to judge the patient's worth but are simply numbers that help both patient and practitioner know what to do; use words such as *monitor* or *check*, rather than *test*.

- Provide information about how to use the results to make proactive decisions or adjustments and when or how often to contact the provider to review readings.

- Help patients identify and address barriers to monitoring. Ask patients to identify behavioral and psychosocial issues they are likely to encounter. For example:

  - How will you handle monitoring in public places or various social situations? How will you handle monitoring at work? How will you handle questions in these situations?

  - What kind of support would you like from your family and friends? Do you want them to ask you about your results or wait until you tell them?

  - How will you handle it when you are working hard and your results do not reflect your efforts?

- Let patients know you understand that it is frustrating to do the same thing one day to the next and have very different results.

- Stress that there is no such thing as perfection in blood glucose levels. The patient's values are what count the most in most situations.

Blood Glucose Meters

A variety of blood glucose meters are available with differing capabilities. The size of the blood sample needed ranges from 0.3 µL to 10.0 µL, depending on the meter. Most meters have memory capability for storing variable amounts of data, and many have relatively sophisticated data management software that enables the user to enter medication/insulin dosages, carbohydrate intake, and exercise. Some meters can be downloaded using software programs that provide data analysis (blood glucose averages, percent of readings within the target range, etc.). You can use these software programs to download data at the time of the visit. Because patients frequently do not utilize the data management

When Patients' Blood Glucose Logbooks Are Inaccurate

Studies have shown that patients often add, delete, or alter numbers in their glucose log books. While some of these inaccuracies are likely due to simple recording errors or represent the patient's estimate of their blood glucose, others are deliberately fabricated or changed.

Fear is the most likely underlying cause of this common occurrence. It is human nature to want others to think well of us. Therefore, making the frequency of testing or the results look better than they are often reflects the patients' desire to have us think well of them or their diabetes self-management efforts.

An effective strategy to prevent this from happening is to ask the patient what they think of their glucose readings rather than telling the patient what you think. In addition, teach patients:

- That blood glucose readings are information used by both of you to make decisions, not a judgment of their efforts or worth as a person;

- How to use the information to make the many daily decisions that are needed to manage diabetes effectively and to make adjustments in their medications or other therapies;

- How you will use the information during a visit;

- How to incorporate monitoring into their daily routine, solve problems, and obtain family support.

capabilities of their meters, they should be encouraged to keep a handwritten logbook.

All meters have a toll-free number on the back that patients can call for technical assistance. Most meter companies also have user-friendly Web sites. Whereas blood glucose meters are generally covered by insurance, the number of test strips covered may be limited.

A variety of meters are available that can be used for alternate-site testing, which is reportedly less painful than fingertip testing. Alternate sites include the forearm, the palm of the hand, and the thigh. Blood glucose levels documented via alternate-site testing tend to lag behind fingertip levels. Alternate-site testing should not be used when blood glucose levels are changing rapidly, such as after meals or exercise, or when hypoglycemia is suspected.

All meters are plasma referenced; that is, a fingerstick (capillary) sample should be comparable to a simultaneously obtained venous sample performed in a laboratory. Technique and meter accuracy should be assessed regularly, especially if hemoglobin A1C values do not correlate with self-monitoring blood glucose readings. During initial training and periodic reassessments, patients should be asked to demonstrate their self-monitoring technique.

How can I help patients choose a blood glucose meter?

Many insurance companies dictate which meter a patient can use regardless of the needs and abilities of the patient. Whenever possible, however, patients should consider their preferences, technical abilities, and physical limitations when choosing a meter. For example, very small meters or meters with very small strips can be difficult to use for people with visual impairment or problems with manual dexterity. Some meter displays may be more difficult to read than others. In addition, some patients may be intimidated by overly complicated meters and may be less likely to use such a meter.

Recording Blood Glucose Results

Keeping a written logbook that is updated with every self-monitored blood glucose reading allows patients to get immediate feedback about their treatment regimen and their self-management decisions. This is especially important for patients using basal/bolus insulin therapy, who need to make daily adjustments in their pre-meal insulin dosages. Most meter companies provide logbooks to providers and patients. By going to a manufacturer's Web site, patients can find out how to obtain additional logbooks. Many Web sites also offer a free, downloadable logbook. Some patients prefer to develop their own logbooks by using a spreadsheet format.

Meters with memory and download capabilities have nearly caused the extinction of handwritten logbooks. Unfortunately, however, most patients do not review the meter memory or download the data often enough—if at all—to make timely treatment adjustments. Even though memory meters can store many blood glucose readings and the meter downloads can provide sophisticated analyses of blood glucose trends, entering blood glucose readings by hand is generally more helpful for using the information. This method gives patients the opportunity to assess their blood glucose levels daily or weekly. Handwritten logbooks also permit easy entry of other important data, including medication dosages, carbohydrate intake, and exercise.

- Patients who do not keep handwritten records need guidelines for how often to download the meter and how to interpret the data from these downloads.

- Software programs are available for patients and practitioners to use to download data from selected meters and perform trend analysis.

What do my patients need to know about their blood glucose meters?

Some tips you can share with patients about their blood glucose meters include:

- Patients need to know technical aspects of using their meter and how to solve meter-related problems. Point out the toll-free hotline number on the back of the meter.

- Availability of reimbursement for strips and meters is another issue. If none is available, ask if paying for a meter and strips is a problem.

- Remember to point out where to get help choosing a meter (e.g., from a diabetes educator or pharmacist) if one is not prescribed by an insurance or managed care plan.

Hemoglobin A1C

Hemoglobin A1C measures nonreversible glycosylation of the hemoglobin molecule. The rate of formation of hemoglobin A1C is directly related to blood glucose concentration and reflects a time-weighted mean of the patient's blood glucose level over the previous 2 to 3 months. Hemoglobin A1C is predictive of the risk for micro- and macrovascular complications.

Slightly differing hemoglobin A1C goals have been established by the ADA and the AACE; however, as with blood glucose goals, hemoglobin A1C goals must be individualized for patient safety. Our recommendations are as follows:

- A1C goal: ≤7.0%, individualized for patient safety

- A1C testing interval: twice annually in stable patients; four or more times per year if glycemic control is not achieved or if treatment changes

The evidence for the importance of achieving blood glucose levels that are as close to normal as possible in older adults with diabetes is overwhelming. However, it is less clear what the target A1C levels should be for older adults with a recent diagnosis of diabetes. In other words, an older adult with a recent diagnosis has a far lower risk of developing complications over his or her lifetime than does someone whose diagnosis was made when he or she was much younger. Some geriatrics groups thus argue that for older adults with a recent diagnosis of diabetes, the A1C targets do not have to be as stringent.

The A1C level is used in assessing the overall effectiveness of the treatment regimen and in adjusting the regimen to improve glycemic control. The ability to obtain in-office, point-of-care hemoglobin A1C measurements has been shown to improve glycemic control by providing immediate feedback on the adequacy of the current treatment regimen. Timely adjustments to the regimen, based on out-of-range hemoglobin A1C values, can be made at the time of the next visit. This facilitates communication between you and patients about regimen changes and encourages a collaborative relationship in which patients actively participate in their diabetes management.

The A1C goals cited by organizations such as the ADA are based on pay-for-performance metrics that include the frequency of testing A1C and the percentage of patients not at their goal. The goals for hemoglobin A1C management listed in the Ambulatory Care Quality Alliance (AQA) starter set of performance measures for diabetes are as follows:

- Management—Percentage of patients with diabetes with one or more A1C test(s) conducted during the measurement year

- Control—Percentage of patients with diabetes with most recent A1C level >9.0% (poor control)

Hemoglobin A1C values should correlate with self-monitoring blood glucose results. The data correlating A1C with serum blood glucose in **Table 6-1** were derived from quarterly, 7-point self-monitoring blood glucose profiles (pre- and post-meal, at bedtime, and at 3 AM) of the Diabetes Control and Complications Trial (DCCT) cohort. The self-monitoring blood glucose average in patients measuring blood glucoses less frequently than these intervals may not correlate with the A1C values listed in the table.

Table 6-1. Correlating A1C with Serum Blood Glucose

Hemoglobin A1C	Mean Blood Glucose
6%	135 mg/dL
7%	170 mg/dL
8%	205 mg/dL
9%	240 mg/dL
10%	275 mg/dL
11%	310 mg/dL
12%	345 mg/dL

Data from: American Diabetes Association. Standards of medical care in diabetes—2006. Diabetes Care. 2006;29 Suppl 1:S4-42. [PMID: 16373931]

When A1C levels are higher than expected, given the self-monitoring blood glucose results, consider the following possibilities:

- Blood glucose levels that are outside the target range at times when self-monitoring blood glucose is not being done (e.g., postprandially or overnight)

- Technical problem with the blood glucose meter or strips or faulty technique

- Inaccurate data recorded in patient's logbook (If possible, use meter download or review meter memory to confirm.)

- Hemoglobinopathy or anemia (because A1C is influenced by blood loss and rapid red blood cell turnover)

What do my patients need to know about their A1C results?

When reviewing A1C results with patients, the following points are important to include in the discussion:

- Tell them that the results reflect their blood glucose levels over the past 2 to 3 months.

- Explain what their results mean in relationship to recommended target levels. Phrases such as *out of the target range* are more meaningful than *out of control*.

- Point out the importance of these results as a way of understanding their risk for the complications of diabetes.

- Explain what the A1C results mean in relationship to blood glucose levels. (Again, use Table 6-1 as a guide.)

- Emphasize that the results are not a "report card" of their efforts or yours. The A1C is simply additional information to help develop an effective treatment program.

Fructosamine

Fructosamine (glycosylated protein) levels reflect average blood glucose values over the previous 1 to 2 weeks. These levels are used less frequently than hemoglobin A1C levels but can be useful in situations in which hemoglobin A1C measurement is not reliable (e.g., hemolytic anemia).

7. Oral Diabetes Drugs

The combination of progressive beta-cell dysfunction and increasing insulin resistance leads to the need for pharmacologic therapy to control hyperglycemia in most patients with type 2 diabetes. The United Kingdom Prospective Diabetes Study (UKPDS) showed that fewer than 25% of persons treated with diet and exercise were able to maintain hemoglobin A1C levels of <7% after 3 years, and fewer than 10% achieved this goal after 9 years.

The goal of pharmacotherapy is to achieve target hemoglobin A1C and fasting and postprandial glucose values within a few months. This is achievable if medications are prescribed early and at adequate dosages. The two major categories of oral diabetes drugs are insulin secretagogues and insulin sensitizers that enhance insulin action. Information about oral hypoglycemic drugs is provided in **Table 7-1.**

When does a patient need to start oral therapy?

If the fasting plasma glucose level remains greater than 126 mg/dL or the hemoglobin A1C value remains above 7% after lifestyle changes (medical nutrition therapy and exercise) have been in place for 4 to 6 weeks, pharmacologic therapy with an oral agent should be initiated.

What do I need to teach my patients about oral medications?

- At the initial visit, describe the progressive nature of type 2 diabetes and stress that oral medications are part of the continuum of care for many patients with diabetes. These agents should *not* be characterized as a sign of patient failure or an indication that the diabetes is worse.

- Provide written information about the medication name, dosage, and timing with food intake and when to take the medication for maximum effectiveness.

- Because of financial or other concerns, many patients choose to take one of their oral medications but not others. Therefore, stress the action and synergistic nature of multiple medications.

- Ask that patients contact you about side effects rather than stopping the medication.

- Provide instructions on how to handle forgotten and missed doses.

- Ask patients to get a first-alert bracelet because of potential hypoglycemia and hyperglycemia issues.

- Provide patients with *Keeping Track of Your Pills* in Chapter 7 of the *Diabetes Care Guide Toolkit* to help them remember to take their medications and *Your Wallet-Sized Medical Record* (in the same chapter of the toolkit) to keep a record of their physician's name, their medical conditions, any allergies they have, and their medications. (Remind them that because the latter tool will contain confidential information, they should be careful who has access to it.)

Insulin Secretagogues

Insulin secretagogues stimulate pancreatic secretion of insulin, which in turn decreases hepatic glucose production and enhances the uptake of glucose by muscle. There are two classes of secretagogues: sulfonylureas and non-sulfonylurea secretagogues.

Sulfonylureas

- *Mechanism of action*: Stimulate insulin secretion from the pancreas.

Table 7-1. Oral Hypoglycemic Drugs

Drug	Duration	Comments
Secretagogues: Sulfonylureas—1st generation		These medications have been largely replaced by 2nd generation sulfonylureas. Because they are cleared hepatically, these medications should be avoided in patients with abnormal liver function.
Tolbutamide	10–12 hours	
Tolazamide	12–24 hours	
Chloropropamide	>24 hours	
Secretagogues: Sulfonylureas—2nd generation		Consider using in patients starting oral therapy who have normal hepatic/renal function and in patients already on an insulin sensitizer who need additional glucose lowering. Avoid using in patients with impaired renal function (creatinine clearance <60 mL/min) or who are elderly. There is a risk of hypoglycemia for those who skip meals.
Glyburide	12–24 hours	
Glipizide	12–24 hours	
Glimepiride	24 hours	
Nonsulfonylurea secretagogues		Consider using in patients with modest postprandial hyperglycemia and in patients who have irregular timing of meals. These agents can be used in patients with renal impairment.
Repaglinide	4–6 hours	
Nateglinide	4 hours	
Biguanides		Good first-line agent for overweight or obese patients. Consider using in patients already on a secretagogue who need additional glucose lowering. Avoid in patients with renal or hepatic impairment or New York Heart Association (NYHA) class III or IV heart failure.
Metformin	12–18 hours	
Metformin extended release	24 hours	
Alpha-glucosidase inhibitors		Consider using in patients who have primarily postprandial hyperglycemia. Avoid in patients with gastrointestinal disease or hepatic or renal insufficiency. May be used in combination with sensitizers or sulfonylurea secretagogues but not nonsulfonylurea secretagogues.
Acarbose	2–3 hours	
Miglitol	2–3 hours	
Thiazolidinediones		These agents are used as monotherapy in patients on a secretagogue or metformin. Avoid in patients with abnormal hepatic function or NYHA class III or IV heart failure. They may cause weight gain and/or peripheral edema.
Rosiglitazone	Days–weeks	
Pioglitazone	Days–weeks	
Dipeptidyl peptidase IV inhibitors		This drug is used as monotherapy or in conjunction with metformin or thiazolidinediones in patients with type 2 diabetes for whom diet and exercise or their current drug regimen is insufficient as treatment.
Sitagliptin	24 hours	

- *Dosing*: Typically dosed twice daily with the exception of glimepiride, which is taken once daily. The maximum effective dosage of sulfonylureas is usually half the maximum dosage listed on the package insert.

- *Efficacy*: Lower fasting and postprandial glucose levels. Lower A1C value by to 1 to 2 percentage points.

- *Benefits*: The UKPDS showed a 25% decrease in microvascular complications and a 12% reduction in all diabetes-related endpoints in patients who were treated with sulfonylureas, with or without insulin.

- *Adverse effects*: Can cause weight gain and hypoglycemia. These medications are metabolized by the liver and cleared by the kidney (with the exception of glimepiride, which is excreted both renally and hepatically) and should therefore be used cautiously in patients with impaired hepatic or renal function. Glyburide has an active metabolite and can cause prolonged hypoglycemia in cases of renal failure. Sulfonylureas should be used at low dosages in the elderly, who may have a decreased glomerular filtration rate even with a normal serum creatinine concentration. Caution should also be used with patients who tend to skip meals, as these medications stimulate insulin secretion in a glucose-independent manner.

Nonsulfonylurea Secretagogues

• *Mechanism of action*: Rapidly stimulate insulin secretion from the pancreas.

• *Dosing*: Taken before meals. If a meal is skipped, the medication is not taken.

• *Efficacy*: Lower postprandial blood sugar. Lower A1C by 0.5 to 2 percentage points.

• *Benefits*: Rapid onset of action and short duration of action. Lower risk of hypoglycemia and less weight gain compared with sulfonylureas. Repaglinide is cleared hepatically and may be used in patients with renal impairment. A good option for patients who have erratic timing of meals.

• *Adverse effects*: Metabolized by the liver so should be used with caution in patients with impaired hepatic function.

Insulin Sensitizers

Agents that enhance insulin action work through several mechanisms. They may inhibit glucose absorption, inhibit hepatic gluconeogenesis and glycogenolysis, or increase glucose uptake in fat and muscle. These medications fall into three categories: biguanides (metformin),

thiazolidinediones (TZDs), and alpha-glucosidase inhibitors.

Biguanides (Metformin)

• *Mechanism of action*: Inhibits hepatic gluconeogenesis and to a lesser extent glycogenolysis. Also enhances insulin sensitivity in muscle and fat.

• *Dosing*: Typically given twice daily in divided doses (breakfast and supper). Can be given three times daily with meals. The extended form can be given once daily.

• *Efficacy*: Lowers the level of fasting and postprandial blood sugars. Lowers A1C value by 1 to 2 percentage points.

• *Benefits*: Does not cause hypoglycemia when used as monotherapy and can cause weight loss. Macrovascular benefits: In the UKPDS, the risk of a myocardial infarction decreased by 39% among overweight patients treated with metformin. Diabetes prevention: A 31% reduced incidence of diabetes occurred among persons with impaired glucose tolerance who were treated with metformin in the Diabetes Prevention Program (DPP).

• *Adverse effects*: Lactic acidosis is a rare but potentially fatal adverse effect of metformin. The risk of lactic acidosis is increased if baseline renal function is abnormal or if an acute insult is affecting the kidneys, such as dehydration, major surgery, chronic heart failure, or administration of radiocontrast agents (e.g., during computed tomographic scanning or cardiac catheterization). Metformin should not be prescribed if the serum creatinine is >1.5 mg/dL in men or >1.4 mg/dL in women. Twenty-four hour creatinine clearance should be assessed in the elderly (age >80 years) prior to prescribing metformin. The renal clearance of metformin is decreased approximately 30% when the creatinine clearance is below 60 mL/min. Additional side effects include nausea, abdominal pain or cramping, diarrhea, and a metallic taste. Starting with a small dosage followed by dosage escalation can minimize these side effects.

Thiazolidinediones

- *Mechanism of action*: Enhance insulin sensitivity in muscle and fat by increasing the expression of glucose transporters.

- *Dosing*: Taken once or twice daily.

- *Efficacy*: Lower the level of fasting and post-prandial blood sugar. Lower A1C values by 1 to 2 percentage points. Typically, 8 to 12 weeks are needed to achieve maximum therapeutic effect, and the effects taper over weeks after the medication is discontinued.

- *Benefits*: Do not cause hypoglycemia when used as monotherapy. Salutary effect on lipid parameters: lower the level of triglycerides, raise the HDL cholesterol level, and increase the LDL cholesterol particle size. Reduce levels of inflammatory cytokines associated with cardiovascular risk and may improve endothelial dysfunction.

- *Adverse effects*: Can cause modest to significant weight gain, largely because of fluid retention, and may also cause peripheral edema. These effects are generally less pronounced at lower dosages. These medications should be avoided in patients with New York Heart Association functional class III or IV heart failure. The agent troglitazone was withdrawn from U.S. market due to hepatotoxicity. The U.S. Food and Drug Administration (FDA) no longer issues a black box warning to regularly monitor the levels of transaminases in persons taking pioglitazone or rosiglitazone; however, baseline transaminase levels should be checked before these medications are started. If these levels are >2.5 times normal, these agents should not be used.

Alpha-Glucosidase Inhibitors

- *Mechanism of action*: Competitively block the enzyme alpha-glucosidase in the brush borders of the small intestine, resulting in absorption of carbohydrates in the mid and distal small intestine (delayed absorption).

- *Dosing:* Taken before meals that contain carbohydrates. If a meal is skipped, the medication is not taken.

- *Efficacy*: Lower postprandial hyperglycemia. Lower A1C values by 0.5 to 1 percentage points.

- *Benefits:* Macrovascular disease: The Study to Prevent Non–Insulin-Dependent Diabetes Mellitus (STOP-NIDDM) trial showed a nearly 50% reduction in the incidence of cardiovascular events among persons with impaired glucose tolerance who were treated with acarbose.

- *Adverse effects*: Should not be used in people with severe hepatic or renal impairment or in those with gastrointestinal disease. Gastrointestinal side effects can be severe and include bloating, abdominal cramps, diarrhea, and flatulence.

Novel Therapies—Dipeptidyl Peptidase IV Inhibitors

These oral medications inhibit dipeptidyl peptidase IV (DPP IV)—the enzyme that degrades endogenously secreted incretins, including glucagon-like peptide-1 and glucose-dependent insulinotropic polypeptide. Higher levels of these incretin hormones lead to increased insulin secretion and suppression of glucagon secretion. Sitagliptin (Januvia) was the first DPP IV inhibitor to be approved by the FDA for use as monotherapy or in combination with metformin or TZDs. A decision from the FDA regarding approval of vildagliptin, another DPP IV inhibitor, is expected in 2007 (after publication of the *ACP Diabetes Care Guide*).

Sitagliptin

- *Mechanism of action:* Inhibits degradation of DPP IV, leading to increased insulin secretion and decreased glucagon secretion.

- *Dosing:* 100 mg taken once daily, with or without meals.

- *Efficacy:* Lowers A1C by 0.7%–1.4%. Has a greater effect on postprandial than fasting glucose levels.

- *Benefits:* Is weight neutral. The mechanism of action involves glucose-dependent insulin secretion. When used as monotherapy or in combination with insulin sensitizers (metformin or TZDs), this drug does not cause hypoglycemia.

- *Adverse effects:* Metabolized in the liver but excreted largely unchanged in the urine. Dosage needs to be reduced by 50% to 75% in patients with renal insufficiency. Most common adverse effects include nasopharyngitis and headache.

How should I choose an agent for a patient starting oral therapy?

Consider whether a patient is relatively more insulin deficient or insulin resistant when choosing an initial oral agent. Persons with central obesity, even those who are only modestly overweight, are typically insulin resistant. Insulin sensitizers are a good choice for initial pharmacotherapy for these patients: for example, metformin 500 mg once or twice daily or a TZD at the lowest dosage, depending on the degree of hyperglycemia when pharmacotherapy is started.

Sulfonylureas may be used in combination with insulin sensitizers when pharmacotherapy is started if significant hyperglycemia (A1C value >9%) and concern about starting a sensitizer at a higher dosage are factors. Lean persons tend to be relatively more insulin deficient than resistant and may benefit less from insulin

sensitizers. For them, it is reasonable to try a sulfonylurea with the understanding that if that fails, insulin treatment will most likely be needed. Some persons have primarily postprandial hyperglycemia without significantly elevated fasting blood sugar levels. In them, it is reasonable to consider either an alpha-glucosidase inhibitor or a nonsulfonylurea secretagogue at meals.

A major problem with diabetes management is that physicians too often start patients on an initial low dosage of a sensitizer or secretagogue and fail to titrate the medication after a few months, despite no improvement in glycemic control. Inertia on the part of physicians to start and accelerate pharmacotherapy leads to suboptimal treatment of hyperglycemia. For example, after the initial 3 months of pharmacotherapy, if the A1C value decreases from 9% to 8.3%, physicians will too often "leave things alone" and recheck laboratory values in another 3 to 6 months. Clinician inertia can leave patients with A1C values above target for months or years. Starting pharmacotherapy is just the first step, and active management with medication titration should be pursued by both the patient and the physician.

Starting, Titrating, and Adding Oral Agents

The natural history of type 2 diabetes includes progressive beta-cell failure and insulin resistance. Increasing the dosages of existing medications and adding new classes of medications are generally the rule for patients with type 2 diabetes: the UKPDS showed that more than 70% of patients fail to maintain a hemoglobin A1C value below 7% with diet or one oral agent.

The dosage of an oral agent should be increased every 4 to 8 weeks until fasting and postprandial glucose levels are at target. You can base these adjustments on home monitoring values you obtain by calling patients between visits. After 3 months, plasma glucose and hemoglobin A1C levels should be measured. If these levels continue to be elevated, the dosage of the initial oral agent should again be increased and/or a second oral agent with a complementary mechanism of action should be added. It is not always necessary to titrate a medication to its maximal dosage before starting a second agent. Increasing the dosage of a sulfonylurea above half the maximum recommended dosage provides little additional therapeutic benefit. Similarly, patients taking 2000 mg of metformin daily are unlikely to get much additional benefit from increasing the dosage to 2550 mg/d (the maximum recommended dosage).

Combination therapy can generally lower the hemoglobin A1C by an additional 0.6 to 2.0 percentage points. The FDA has approved several combinations of oral agents:

- A sulfonylurea with metformin, a TZD, or an alpha-glucosidase inhibitor

- A nonsulfonylurea secretagogue with metformin

- Metformin with a TZD or an alpha-glucosidase inhibitor

Several of these are available as combination products. These may be helpful to reduce the number of pills a patient needs to take; however, dosing and titration options are less flexible with combination products.

Special considerations in prescribing oral diabetes drugs are summarized in **Table 7-2.**

Helping Patients Succeed with Oral Therapy

What facts about each oral medication do my patients need to know?

Sulfonylureas:

- How to prevent, recognize, and treat hypoglycemia.

Table 7-2. Special Considerations When Prescribing Oral Diabetes Drugs

Elderly patients (age >80 years): Sulfonylureas can cause prolonged hypoglycemia in elderly patients, primarily because of renal insufficiency or the skipping of meals; glyburide in particular should be used with caution in elderly patients because it is cleared renally and has an active metabolite. Metformin should be used with caution in elderly patients and avoided if creatinine clearance is abnormal (<60 mL/min).

Renal impairment (creatinine clearance <60 mL/min): Metformin and alpha-glucosidase inhibitors should be avoided. Glyburide dose should be lowered.

Hepatic impairment: Thiazolidinediones and metformin should be avoided.

Congestive heart failure (decompensated or New York Heart Association class III or IV): Thiazolidinediones and metformin should be avoided.

Pregnancy: No oral drugs are approved by the Food and Drug Administration (FDA) for use in pregnancy. NPH insulin, regular insulin, and the rapid-acting insulin analogues aspart and lispro are endorsed by the American Diabetes Association (ADA) for use in pregnancy but are not formally approved by the FDA. Glulisine, the third available short-acting insulin analogue, has not been studied in pregnancy and is not endorsed by the ADA. Similarly, neither of the long-acting insulin analogues (glargine and detemir) has been studied or endorsed by the ADA for use during pregnancy.

- May cause weight gain. Refer for medical nutrition therapy if this is a concern for the patient.

Nonsulfonylurea secretagogues:

- Greatest effect is on postprandial glucose levels.

- Take just before or up to 30 minutes prior to meals. If meal is omitted, do not take medication.

- How to prevent, recognize and treat hypoglycemia.

Metformin:

- Greatest effect is on fasting blood glucose levels.

- Take with largest meal (usually supper) to reduce nausea and metallic taste.

- Can cause weight loss.

- Diarrhea is common but should decrease with time. If diarrhea persists, may need to reduce the dosage or switch to another medication.

- When to discontinue for surgical or contrast dye procedures.

TZDs:

- May take 2 to 12 weeks to become effective, so be patient.

- Fluid retention may cause swelling and modest weight gain (edema).

- Blood tests need to be done as prescribed to monitor liver function.

- When used with a sulfonylurea or insulin, may necessitate a lower dosage of those agents.

Alpha-glucosidase inhibitors:

- Take with the first bite of your meal.

- If you skip a meal, do not take this medication.

- Main side effects are bloating, gas, and diarrhea.

Sitagliptin

- Is weight neutral.

- In patients with renal insufficiency, dosage reduction is necessary.

What should I ask my patients about their oral medications at each visit?

Some questions to ask patients at each visit about their oral medications include:

- Are you having any side effects?

- Are you having trouble paying for any of your medications?

- About how often do you miss taking your medications?

- Are you taking any vitamins or herbal or natural products?

- Do you have difficulty taking your medications? What specific problems have you encountered? How have you tried to solve this problem? What other options do you think may be effective?

- How well do you think your treatment plan is working to manage your diabetes?

- Do you have any questions about your medications?

- How can I help most?

What tips can I provide to help patients remember to take oral medications?

The following tips can be shared with patients to help them remember to take their medications:

- Take at the same time each day.

- Take when you do other routine activities (e.g., eat meals, get ready for bed).

- Store in a pill container with days of the week (see *Keeping Track of Your Pills* in Chapter 7 of the toolkit).

- Keep a dose in a purse, briefcase, or pocket.

- Create a reminder system for doses that are especially hard to remember—for example, a watch with an alarm clock, an electronic reminder through your computer at work, or a sticky note where you will be sure to see it at the appropriate time.

8. Insulins and New Injectables

When does a patient with type 2 diabetes need to be started on insulin?

Indications for insulin in type 2 diabetes are listed below:

- Presence of severe symptoms (such as polydipsia, polyuria, or weight loss), marked hyperglycemia (fasting plasma glucose level >350 mg/dL), or ketonuria at diagnosis or during the course of the disease

- Diabetic ketoacidosis or a hyperosmolar state

- Ineffectiveness of oral agents alone to maintain glucose levels within the patient's target range

- If oral agents are contraindicated

- During pregnancy (and, ideally, prior to conception)

What do I need to teach my patients about insulin?

Some essential points to share with patients about insulin follow:

- In type 1 diabetes, insulin is necessary to sustain life.

- Type 2 diabetes is a progressive disease, and insulin is part of the continuum of care for most patients. Taking insulin is not a sign of patient or provider failure or evidence that the diabetes is worse.

- Diabetes is not a "sugar problem" but a disease of absolute insulin deficiency (type 1) or relative insulin deficiency and insulin resistance (type 2). The injection or inhalation of insulin is the only way to treat type 1 diabetes and the most natural and effective method for replacing this essential hormone in type 2 diabetes that no longer responds to other treatments.

- Provide written information about the name of the insulin, the dosage, the timing with food and exercise, peak times, and possible drug interactions.

- Hypoglycemia prevention, symptoms, and treatment; managing insulin dosing during an acute illness; and the need for diabetes identification are essential components of education for patients taking insulin.

- Discuss a plan for contacting you about hypoglycemia (e.g., any severe episodes, more than two events per week) and hyperglycemia.

- Food intake and activity may need to be adjusted to prevent weight gain.

- Discuss how to handle forgotten and missed doses.

- Inform patients that exercise increases insulin sensitivity and, hence, that adjustments to insulin are often required when exercise is undertaken.

Types of Insulin

The goal of insulin therapy is to mimic normal physiologic insulin secretion as closely as possible. Normal insulin consists of low levels of basal insulin secreted at all times to regulate hepatic glucose production overnight and between meals. At mealtimes, nutrient ingestion stimulates an acute, first-phase secretion of insulin followed by a second secretion phase that lasts for as long as blood glucose levels are elevated. Mealtime insulin dynamics inhibit hepatic glucose production and promote glucose disposal, maintaining glucose levels within the normal range until they return to pre-meal levels. As this occurs, insulin secretion also decreases to basal concentrations.

Insulins available for clinical use can be categorized as basal insulins or prandial insulins. Insulins used for basal requirements are long-acting and intermediate-acting insulins. These include insulin glargine, insulin detemir, and neutral protamine Hagedorn (NPH) insulin. (The latter is an intermediate-acting insulin that has both basal and prandial characteristics in that it peaks about 4–8 hours after administration.) Insulins used for prandial requirements are the rapid-acting insulin analogues (insulin lispro, insulin aspart, and insulin glulisine) and short-acting regular insulin.

Premixed insulins can be used to provide both basal and prandial requirements. Premixed insulins are either human insulin mixtures (containing NPH and regular insulin) or insulin analogue mixtures. Premixed insulins include those listed below.

- 70/30 insulin (70% NPH and 30% regular)

- 50/50 insulin (50% NPH and 50% regular)

- Humalog mix 75/25—contains 75% neutral protamine lispro (NPL), which has similar pharmacokinetic properties to NPH insulin, and 25% lispro (Humalog)

- Humalog mix 50/50—contains 50% NPL and 50% lispro (Humalog)

- NovoLog mix 70/30—contains 70% neutral protamine aspart, which has similar pharmacokinetic properties to NPH insulin, and 30% aspart (NovoLog)

Insulin preparations that are currently available in the United States are shown in **Table 8-1**. Insulins are either recombinant human insulin products or insulin analogues. Pork and beef insulins are no longer sold in the United States. The rapid-acting analogues are generally preferred to regular insulin because their pharmacodynamic properties are more physiologic and are associated with less intersite and intrasite variability in absorption (between different sites and at the same site when injected on different days). Similarly, basal insulin analogues are less variable than NPH insulin.

In January 2006, the U.S. Food and Drug Administration (FDA) approved a powdered insulin formulation for administration via the pulmonary route. The pharmacokinetics of insulin administered via inhalation are similar to those of the rapid-acting insulin analogues, and thus this formulation is suitable for prandial use. Additionally, clinical trials have shown that inhaled insulin is as effective as subcutaneously administered insulin, and many patients prefer it. Inhaled insulin use is associated with a clinically insignificant increase in the titer of nonneutralizing insulin antibodies but no significant change in pulmonary function when compared with subcutaneously administered insulin. However, pulmonary function testing should be performed prior to starting a patient on inhaled insulin, 6 months after starting the insulin, and at least annually thereafter. Inhaled insulin is contraindicated in patients with chronic obstructive pulmonary disease and in those who smoke or who have smoked within 6 months. It is not contraindicated in patients with stable asthma.

Insulin Regimens for Type 2 Diabetes

In patients with type 2 diabetes, the addition of a basal insulin is often the first step in initiating insulin treatment. In this situation, oral agents (sensitizers and/or secretagogues) are usually continued at the same dosage.

If postprandial glucose levels remain elevated despite normalization of fasting glucose levels, the addition of a prandial insulin is recommended. Once a patient with type 2 diabetes requires prandial insulin, oral insulin secretagogues can be stopped, but insulin sensitizers should be continued in obese, insulin-resistant persons.

Basal Insulin Only

The early use of insulin when oral agents are ineffective can prevent months or years of ongoing suboptimal blood glucose control. In the

Table 8-1. Currently Available Insulin Preparations

Insulin	Manufacturer	Onset	Peak	Duration
Rapid-acting (insulin analogues)				
Insulin lispro (Humalog)	Eli Lilly	<15 minutes	1–2 hours	3–4 hours
Insulin aspart (NovoLog)	Novo Nordisk	<15 minutes	1–2 hours	3–5 hours
Insulin glulisine (Apidra)	Sanofi-Aventis	10–30 minutes	0.5–3 hours	3–5 hours
Inhaled insulin powder				
Exubera	Pfizer	10–20 minutes	2 hours	Up to 6 hours
Short-acting				
Humulin regular	Eli Lilly	0.5–1 hour	2–4 hours	3–6 hours
Novolin regular	Novo Nordisk	0.5–1 hour	2–4 hours	Up to 8 hours
Intermediate-acting				
Humulin NPH	Eli Lilly	2–4 hours	4–10 hours	10–16 hours
Novolin NPH	Novo Nordisk	2–4 hours	4–10 hours	10–16 hours
Long-acting				
Insulin glargine (Lantus)	Sanofi-Aventis	2–4 hours	Peakless	20–24 hours
Insulin detemir (Levemir)	Novo Nordisk	1–2 hours	Minimal or 2–12 hours*	Up to 24 hours (dose dependent)
Human insulin mixtures				
70% NPH/30% regular				
Humulin 70/30	Eli Lilly	0.5–2 hours	2–10 hours	10–16 hours
Novolin 70/30	Novo Nordisk	0.5–2 hours	2–10 hours	10–16 hours
50% NPH/50% regular				
Humulin 50/50	Eli Lilly	0.5–2 hours	2–5 hours	10–16 hours
Analogue Mixtures				
75% lisproprotamine/25% lispro (Humalog Mix 75/25)	Eli Lilly	<15 minutes	1–2 hours	10–16 hours
50% lispro protamine/50% lispro (Humalog Mix 50/50)	Eli Lilly	<15 minutes	1–2 hours	10–12 hours
70% aspart protamine/30% aspart (NovoLog Mix 70/30)	Novo Nordisk	<15 minutes	1–2 hours	10–16 hours

Note: The time course of action of each insulin may vary among persons or at different times in the same person. Because of this variation, the time periods indicated here should be considered general guidelines only.

*Varies among references.

Treat-to-Target study, the addition of nighttime basal insulin to oral agents lowered hemoglobin A1C values from 8.6% to 7% in approximately 10 weeks. Moreover, the addition of basal insulin is more cost effective than the addition of a third oral agent.

- Use NPH, glargine, or detemir insulin at bedtime.

- Begin with a dosage of 10 U or 0.1 U/kg.

- Titrate the basal insulin dosage every 3 to 5 days until the fasting glucose level is at goal (usually <120 mg/dL) using the algorithm in **Table 8-2**.

- Continue oral medications (insulin sensitizers and secretagogues) at the same dosage initially.

Premixed Insulin at Supper

A single daily injection of insulin is indicated if fasting glucose and post-supper glucose levels are elevated. Premixed analogues are the preferred type of insulin for this regimen.

- Starting dosage: 10 U or 0.1 U/kg

- Follow a general approach to adjusting insulin dosage in diabetes patients (**Table 8-3**), but ensure that the blood glucose level at bedtime does not drop below 100 mg/dL.

- If bedtime blood glucose goes below 100 mg/dL, the patient should eat a bedtime snack. If blood glucose is persistently below 100 mg/dL at bedtime, the insulin dosage should be adjusted.

Combination Insulin Two or Three Times Daily

If a patient is taking basal insulin at night and the blood glucose level is elevated at lunch and dinner, the basal insulin alone is not sufficient. In this situation, combinations of basal and

Table 8-2. Titrating Basal Insulin*

If Fasting Blood Glucose Level Is:	Increase Insulin Dose by:
121–140 mg/dL	2 U
141–160 mg/dL	4 U
161–180 mg/dL	6 U
>180 mg/dL	8 U

*Starting dose: 10 U or 0.1 U/kg body weight. Titration should stop if blood glucose drops below 70 mg/dL during the night.

prandial insulin should be injected twice (or, occasionally, three times) daily. Typically, a combination of prandial and intermediate (basal) insulin—either premixed or mixed by the patient—is injected before breakfast and before dinner. In patients with nocturnal hypoglycemia, the intermediate-acting insulin should be given at bedtime rather than before dinner, necessitating a third injection and ruling out the use of a premixed insulin. The success of this insulin regimen depends on the consistent intake of carbohydrates at meals and snacks.

- Starting dosage of insulin is approximately 0.6 U/kg daily but may be higher in obese patients because of their increased insulin resistance.

- Traditionally, the dosage of the premixed insulin is divided to provide two thirds of the insulin in the morning and one third in the evening before meals. If the fixed-dosage premixed insulin is not effective, patients may need to mix the individual components of these insulins in individualized combinations (split-mix insulin regimen).

- When split-mix insulin regimens are used, the ratios of prandial and basal insulin are usually initiated as follows:

  - Two thirds of the morning dosage is given as basal insulin (NPH).

  - One third of the morning dosage is given as prandial insulin (rapid-acting analogue or regular insulin).

  - The evening dosage of insulin is split evenly between prandial (rapid-acting or

regular) and basal insulin (NPH). The basal insulin may be given either before supper or at bedtime.

- The insulin dosage is titrated based on blood glucose levels before meals and at bedtime as follows (with corresponding dosage decreases if glucose levels are below target):

  - If fasting glucose is elevated, increase pre-supper (or bedtime) basal insulin.

  - If bedtime glucose is elevated, increase pre-supper prandial insulin.

  - If pre-lunch glucose is elevated, increase morning prandial insulin.

  - If pre-dinner glucose is elevated, increase morning basal insulin.

- Insulin secretagogues should be stopped once regimens containing prandial insulin are instituted. Insulin sensitizers should be continued in obese, insulin-resistant patients.

Basal-Bolus Regimens

This is the most "physiologic" of the insulin regimens and comprises prandial insulin ("bolus") given before each meal and basal insulin given once or twice daily. Although basal-bolus regimens require several injections daily (typically, four injections), they provide more dietary flexibility and allow patients to skip meals or change mealtimes. As with mixed insulin regimens, insulin secretagogues should be stopped when this regimen is begun, but insulin sensitizers may be continued.

- The long-acting insulins (glargine or detemir) are the most commonly used basal insulins in this regimen. The basal insulin is usually taken before bedtime but is sometimes taken before breakfast. Sometimes, it is taken twice daily. NPH insulin may also be used.

- Rapid-acting insulin analogues are recommended as the bolus/prandial insulin and are taken prior to each meal.

Table 8-3. General Approach to Adjusting Insulin Dosage in Diabetes

Problem	Cause	Solution
Fasting hyperglycemia	Not enough basal insulin at bedtime *OR* Too much basal insulin at bedtime (rebound from overnight hypoglycemia)	Check 3 am blood sugar. If high, increase basal insulin at bedtime (NPH or insulin glargine). If low, decrease basal insulin at bedtime.
Pre-lunch hyperglycemia	Not enough rapid acting insulin at breakfast *OR* Not enough morning NPH	Increase amount of rapid-acting insulin at breakfast—adjust correction dose or the insulin-to-carbohydrate ratio *OR* Increase morning NPH.
Pre-supper hyperglycemia	Not enough rapid-acting insulin at lunch *OR* Not enough morning NPH	Increase amount of rapid-acting insulin at lunch—adjust correction dose or the insulin-to-carbohydrate ratio *OR* Increase morning NPH.
Bedtime hyperglycemia	Not enough rapid-acting insulin at supper	Increase amount of rapid-acting insulin at supper—adjust correction dose or insulin-to-carbohydrate ratio.
Fasting or nocturnal hypoglycemia	Too much basal insulin at bedtime	Decrease bedtime NPH or insulin glargine.
Pre-lunch hypoglycemia	Too much rapid-acting insulin at breakfast *OR* Too much morning NPH	Decrease amount of rapid-acting insulin at breakfast *OR* Decrease morning NPH.
Pre-supper or bedtime hypoglycemia	Too much rapid-acting insulin at lunch or supper	Decrease amount of rapid-acting insulin at lunch or supper.

- Starting basal-bolus insulin dose allocation (**Table 8-4**): If glargine or detemir is used as the basal insulin, the starting dosage allocation is 50% of the total daily dose given as basal insulin and the other 50% as prandial insulin divided equally before meals. If NPH is used, 30% of the total daily dose should be given as NPH at bedtime and the other 70% divided equally before meals.

- Dosage adjustments based on blood glucose levels:

  - If post-breakfast or pre-lunch glucose is elevated, increase pre-breakfast prandial insulin.

  - If post-lunch or pre-supper glucose is elevated, increase pre-lunch prandial insulin.

  - If post-supper glucose is elevated, increase pre-supper prandial insulin.

  - If fasting glucose is elevated, increase basal insulin.

- When making dose adjustments based on blood glucose levels, it is important to remember that factors other than the amount of insulin given can affect these levels:

  - Variability in insulin absorption based on the anatomical site: Insulin is usually absorbed faster from abdominal sites than from the arms and legs. This faster absorption will result in an earlier peak and, possibly, a shorter duration of action.

  - Variability of insulin absorption from day to day and from person to person.

  - The carbohydrate content of a meal: The number of grams of carbohydrate consumed at a particular meal should be consistent from day to day unless the patient has learned how to adjust insulin doses based on carbohydrate counting.

  - The fat content of a meal: Fat content can affect the rate of digestion (i.e., high-fat meals take longer to digest), which can lead to a mismatch between the anticipated insulin action and the actual prandial blood glucose excursions.

  - The type of carbohydrates consumed: Simple carbohydrates (e.g., juice) will increase blood glucose levels faster than complex carbohydrates (e.g., whole grains and fruits) will.

Table 8-4. Basal-Bolus Insulin Dose Allocation*

If a long-acting insulin (glargine or detemir) is used as the basal insulin:
- 50% rapid-acting or regular insulin (divided equally) before meals
- 50% long-acting insulin at bedtime

If NPH is used as the basal insulin:
Rapid-acting or regular insulin
- 30% before breakfast
- 20% before lunch
- 20% before dinner

30% NPH at bedtime

*Percentages of doses are based on a percentage of the estimated total daily dose of insulin.

What do I need to teach patients taking multiple daily insulin injections?

Some information to share with patients who take multiple daily injections of insulin follows:

- Because of financial or other concerns, many patients choose to take one of their medications but not others. Stress the action and synergistic nature of insulins with oral medications or the need for both basal and bolus insulins.

- Basal and bolus insulin coverage is needed in order to mimic physiologic insulin secretion by the pancreas as closely as possible. Explain to patients which insulin provides which type of coverage.

- Although more intensive and requiring greater commitment and effort, multiple-injection insulin regimens provide greater flexibility and may result in improved glucose control. Multiple daily insulin regimens require more time to get insulin dosages balanced. Often, a process of trial and error is involved.

- Patients can use pattern management to adjust insulin dosages based on blood glucose levels.

Pattern Management—Fine-Tuning Insulin Regimens

Insulin Correction Dose Adjustments—Basic Carbohydrate Counting

Insulin correction doses are based on the pre-meal blood glucose level and assume consistent carbohydrate intake (basic carbohydrate counting) at each meal. The correction doses do not adjust for the amount of carbohydrates ingested at the meal. The optimal way to employ an insulin correction dose is to add or subtract insulin from the calculated dosage based on the pre-meal glucose level. (**Table 8-5** presents an algorithm for adjusting prandial insulin.) You will need to provide individualized insulin dosage changes based on patients' activity levels and blood glucose readings.

Advanced Carbohydrate Counting

In advanced carbohydrate counting, the prandial insulin dosage is adjusted based on the amount of carbohydrates eaten at the meal and the pre-meal glucose level. The degree of adjustment is determined by the patient's insulin-to-carbohydrate ratio, pre-meal blood glucose level, and pre-meal glucose target. Advanced carbohydrate counting is most commonly used when patients are taking a basal-bolus regimen or are using continuous subcutaneous insulin infusion pumps.

- The *insulin-to-carbohydrate ratio* is the amount of insulin required to "cover" the carbohydrates in a meal; for example, an insulin-to-carbohydrate ratio of 1:15 means that 1 U of insulin should be given for every 15 g of carbohydrates eaten.

- The *sensitivity factor* reflects the decrease in blood glucose caused by 1 U of insulin. A sensitivity factor of 1:50 means that 1 U of insulin given in the fasting or basal state would decrease the blood glucose level by 50 mg/dL.

Table 8-5. Example of an Algorithm for Adjustment of Prandial Insulin

Blood Glucose (mg/dL)	Prandial Insulin Adjustment
<60	Orange juice –33%
60–80	–25%
81–120	Usual dose
121–160	+10%
161–200	+25%
201–240	+33%
>240	+50%

For example, imagine that a patient's pre-meal glucose target is 100 mg/dL, his insulin-to-carbohydrate ratio is 1:15, and his sensitivity factor is 1:50. If the pre-meal glucose level is 150 mg/dL and the patient is going to eat 60 g of carbohydrates, he would inject 5 U of prandial insulin (4 U to cover the amount of carbohydrates eaten and 1 U because the pre-meal glucose is 50 mg/dL above target).

Insulin Pump Therapy

Continuous subcutaneous insulin infusion (CSII) using an insulin pump is a form of intensive insulin therapy that is most commonly used in type 1 diabetes. However, it is becoming a viable treatment option for patients with type 2 diabetes who require insulin and want both greater lifestyle flexibility and improved glycemic control without taking multiple daily insulin injections.

CSII provides physiologic insulin replacement by delivering a continuous, preprogrammed basal rate along with bolus dosages for meals and to correct hyperglycemia. The amount of prandial insulin is usually determined by using insulin-to-carbohydrate ratios and prescribed algorithms for management of prandial glucose levels that are outside the target range.

CSII therapy enables more accurate titration of insulin delivery to match insulin needs, thereby minimizing blood glucose excursions and reducing the likelihood of hypoglycemia. Because only rapid-acting insulins are used in insulin pumps, this approach features less day-to-day variation in insulin absorption and more predictable pharmacokinetics.

CSII therapy should be an option for any insulin-requiring patient who desires improved metabolic control and increased lifestyle flexibility. The pump does not, however, automatically make adjustments to the amount of insulin infused on the basis of sensor readings. Therefore, to successfully use CSII therapy, patients must meet the following requirements:

• Be capable and willing to monitor their blood glucose at least 4 to 6 times daily

• Know how to accurately count carbohydrates

• Be motivated to make frequent insulin dosage adjustments (e.g., before each meal) based on self-monitoring of blood glucose and carbohydrate intake

• Have the manual dexterity to operate the pump

• Have adequate insurance coverage or be able to afford the pump, associated supplies, and monitoring supplies

Patients who may benefit from CSII therapy include those who:

• Have not been able to achieve glycemic goals on an intensified insulin regimen of multiple daily injections

• Have unacceptable rates of hypoglycemia when following insulin injection regimens that combine intermediate or long-acting insulin (NPH, glargine) with prandial insulin

• Have a marked dawn phenomenon

• Have erratic lifestyles (travel, shift work)

Any patient considering the use of an insulin pump should be referred to a diabetologist or an endocrinologist who is experienced in this mode of therapy and who has the requisite staff to provide training and support.

Helping Patients Make the Transition to Insulin

Initiation of insulin treatment in patients with type 2 diabetes is often delayed. Reasons for this are numerous but include reluctance on the part of both the physician and the patient to start insulin. Insulin is regarded by many patients as ineffective or used to treat only "severe diabetes." Patients often feel that they are failures or feel angry, betrayed, anxious, or frightened when told they need insulin. Overcoming such barriers to insulin use—on the part of the physician as well as the patient—leads to more timely initiation of insulin and potentially improved glycemic control.

In patients taking two or more oral agents, the addition of basal insulin when fasting glucose levels are elevated can safely and easily be achieved in the primary care physician's office. In other cases, a one-time referral to an endocrinologist or referral to a diabetes educator can facilitate the move to insulin.

How can I help my patients with type 2 diabetes make the decision to move to insulin?

Prepare the patient from the time of diagnosis by discussing the progressive nature of type 2 diabetes and mentioning that insulin will likely be needed at some point. Never suggest that a patient may be able to avoid insulin as a "reward" for improving blood glucose levels or for being successful with a weight loss or exercise plan.

Assess the patient's concerns regarding insulin so that appropriate information can be provided. Questions to ask may include:

- How satisfied are you with your current blood glucose levels?

- What do you need to know to consider insulin therapy?

- What is your biggest fear about insulin? What problems do you think you will encounter?

- What do you see as the biggest negative to starting insulin? Biggest positive?

- What support do you have for overcoming barriers?

- How faithful do you think you will be in taking your insulin?

- Are you willing to try insulin? If not, what would make you more willing to try it?

How can I help my patients overcome their fears about starting insulin?

The first step is to determine the real cause of the fear. Although patients often say that they are afraid of the pain of injecting the insulin, this is rarely the real reason. Rather than responding to the issue that is first raised, ask "why is that?" until you get to the heart of the problem. Common concerns and tips for addressing relevant issues are outlined in **Table 8-6**.

Although it is tempting to respond to fears with just facts, a facts-only approach is rarely effective. In addition, such responses may cause patients to feel devalued and embarrassed. Instead, statements such as "Would it help to know that I have started many patients on insulin and none have had to have an amputation?" acknowledge the patient's belief without supporting misinformation.

What do patients need to know to initiate insulin therapy?

Education is a critical component of successful insulin initiation and use. Even if the patient has been to a diabetes education program in the past, initiation of insulin therapy often means that additional education can be reimbursed. Key areas to address are listed below.

- How to monitor blood glucose levels and use the information for making decisions

Table 8-6. Assessing and Addressing Common Concerns about Starting Insulin

Common Concerns	Strategies
Fear of needles or pain from injections	Describe/show very fine needles. Encourage patients to insert needle or give a 'dry' shot well before insulin is needed. Offer insulin pens or other devices that hide the needle from view or may be less painful. Point out that injections are less painful than blood glucose self-monitoring fingersticks. Psychological counseling may be indicated.
Fear of hypoglycemia	Describe new insulins, insulin action times. Explain how to limit and/or prevent episodes. Describe differences in risks for hypoglycemia between multiple and less frequent daily injections. Help the patient identify strategies to maintain independence.
Weight gain	Educate the patient about strategies to minimize weight gain (e.g., decrease caloric intake, increase exercise).
Adverse impact on lifestyle (inconvenience, loss of personal freedom)	Discuss multiple injections as a way to increase flexibility. Demonstrate insulin pens or other devices. Assist patient to identify strategies to maintain independence. Offer available resources and support.
Belief that insulin does not work	Discuss insulin as the most natural and effective way to treat diabetes. Review diabetes as a disease of insulin deficiency and not a "sugar problem."
Belief that insulin means diabetes is worse or a more serious disease	Starting with the initial encounter, discuss all options for treatment as a logical progression. Explain that insulin replacement is a logical step in the progression of the disease in terms of insulin resistance and beta cell failure.
Seeing initiation of insulin as a personal failure	Teach initially and review periodically the concept that beta cell failure is progressive. Avoid statements such as "you've failed oral agents." Reframe the statement as "oral agents/your body has failed you." Avoid using insulin as a threat to encourage weight loss and physical activity.
Belief that insulin causes complications	Provide information about your experience with other people with diabetes. Explain that in the largest study of diabetes to date (UKPDS), tight blood glucose control, with oral agents or insulin, reduced heart disease and stroke as well as diabetic eye disease and kidney damage for people with type 2 diabetes.
Will be treated differently by family and friends	Discuss support patient desires and how to ask for what is needed. Include family in education if requested by patient.

Adapted with permission from Funnell MM, Kruger DF, Spencer M. Self-management support for insulin therapy in type 2 diabetes. Diabetes Educ. 2004;30:274-80.

- The basal-bolus concept of diabetes management and which specific medicines the patient uses for each

- How to use a pen or draw up and inject the correct dosage

- How to use pattern management and make anticipatory and compensatory adjustments in medication dosages

- How to prevent, recognize, and treat hypoglycemia

- How to use glucagon

- The importance of wearing and carrying diabetes identification at all times

See *Getting Started with Insulin* in Chapter 8 of the *Diabetes Care Guide Toolkit* for practical tips your patients can use to successfully begin insulin therapy.

Insulin Regimens for Type 1 Diabetes

The ideal regimen for someone with type 1 diabetes is either basal-bolus treatment or an insulin pump with advanced carbohydrate counting. If neither of these regimens is used, the patient should take at least three injections per day: a mixture of prandial and basal (NPH) insulin prior to breakfast, prandial insulin prior to supper, and basal (NPH) insulin at bedtime.

For patients unable to understand or implement advanced carbohydrate counting, then basic carbohydrate counting with a consistent amount of carbohydrates ingested at each meal is recommended.

- The usual starting dosage of insulin for someone with type 1 diabetes is 0.3 to 0.6 U/kg daily. (Note that the starting dosage in patients with type 2 diabetes is generally higher than this because of insulin resistance.)

- Increased dosage requirements occur in adolescence, during pregnancy, and during times of stress or infection.

- Decreased dosage requirements occur during the honeymoon phase of the disease, during periods of increased physical activity, and during the immediate postpartum period.

Although fine-tuning an insulin regimen is highly individualized for every patient, some glycemic patterns are commonly seen. Refer back to Table 8-3 for a general approach to adjusting insulin in patients with type 1 or type 2 diabetes.

Insulin for Gestational Diabetes

Insulin is indicated in women with gestational diabetes if medical nutrition therapy and exercise alone are insufficient to control fasting and postprandial glucose levels within the target range. The insulin regimen used varies from person to person and depends on which glucose concentrations are elevated. Sometimes, using basal insulin (usually NPH) alone is sufficient; in other situations, both basal and prandial insulins are required.

Helping Patients Succeed With Insulin Therapy

What facts about each insulin do my patients need to know?

Rapid-acting insulin analogues (lispro, aspart, glulisine):

- Take no more than 15 minutes prior to meals to prevent hypoglycemia

- Greatest effect is on postprandial glucose levels

Short-acting (regular) insulin:

- Most effective if taken 30 minutes prior to meals

- Greatest effect is on postprandial glucose levels

Intermediate-acting (NPH) insulin:

- NPH given at night lowers the fasting glucose level; when taken in the morning, its greatest effect is controlling the post-lunch and pre-dinner glucose levels

Long-acting insulin (glargine, detemir):

- Take at about the same time each day

- Do not mix in the same syringe with other insulins

Premixed insulins:

- Not all premixed insulins are the same; do not purchase brands and types other than those that were prescribed

---

What should I ask my patients about their insulin regimens at each visit?

The following questions are helpful for monitoring patients' success and comfort level with their insulin therapy:

• Are you having any problems with high or low blood glucose levels?

• About how often do you miss taking your insulin?

• Do you have difficulty paying for your insulin or any other medications?

• Would you like to learn to adjust your insulin dosage based on your glucose levels or carbohydrate intake?

• Are you having any problems with your insulin? What specific problems have you encountered? What have you tried to solve this problem? What other options do you think may be effective?

• How well do you think your treatment plan is working to manage your diabetes?

• Do you have any questions about your insulin?

• How can I help most?

Can I provide tips to help patients get the most from their insulin?

The following information should be shared with patients to optimize their insulin therapy:

• Take your insulin at the same time each day (unless the patient is on basal-bolus insulin, in which case the insulin is given before meals, whatever time they are eaten).

• Take your insulin when you do other routine activities (e.g., eat meals, get ready for bed).

• Putting off an injection does not make it easier.

• Unopened insulin can be safely stored in the refrigerator until the expiration date.

• Opened vials of insulin can be safely stored at room temperature (less than 30 °C [86 °F]) for 28 to 30 days. If insulin freezes or is exposed to temperatures above 30 °C [86 °F]),

it becomes completely ineffective and must be discarded.

• Insulin pen cartridges have different expiration dates depending on the brand and type of insulin. Follow the manufacturer's instructions.

• Syringes can be safely re-used if handled appropriately: avoid touching the needle and replace the cap over the needle; move the plunger up and down to help prevent clogs; and do not wipe the needle with alcohol, as this removes the silicone coating. Smaller-gauge needles have fewer re-uses than larger-gauge needles before becoming painful.

• Provide information regarding appropriate needle disposal for the patient's community based on local regulations.

New Injectables

In 2005, the FDA approved two new injected drugs for the treatment of diabetes—exenatide (Byetta) and pramlintide (Symlin). Both drugs lower postprandial glucose levels, but they have different clinical applications. **Table 8-7** compares the key considerations of using insulin, exenatide, and pramlintide.

Exenatide

Exenatide is a synthetic form of exendin 4, a naturally occurring hormone that has actions similar to those of glucagon-like peptide type 1 (GLP-1). GLP-1 is an incretin hormone with several actions, including the stimulation of glucose-dependent insulin secretion, the inhibition of glucagon secretion and hepatic glucose production, the delay of gastric emptying, and the suppression of appetite through central pathways that have yet to be elucidated. Endogenous GLP-1 has a half-life of a few minutes and, hence, is not suitable for pharmacologic use, but exenatide, which acts through the GLP-1 receptor, has a longer half-life and can be detected in the circulation 10 hours after administration. The availability of other GLP-1

Table 8-7. Comparison of Insulin, Exenatide, and Pramlintide

Key Considerations	Insulin	Exenatide (Byetta)	Pramlintide (Symlin)
Associated with hypoglycemia	Yes	Yes*	Yes[†]
Associated with weight loss	No	Yes	Yes
Adjust dose for meals or exercise	Yes	No	No
Use with insulin	—	No	Yes
Use with oral agents	Yes	Yes	Yes

*Hypoglycemia can occur when exenatide is used in combination with a sulfonylurea.

[†]Pramlintide potentiates the effects of insulin and therefore can cause potentially severe hypoglycemia. The prandial insulin dose should be reduced by approximately 50% when pramlintide is started.

analogues with different pharmacokinetic properties is expected shortly.

Indications

- FDA approved for use in combination with metformin, sulfonylureas, or both

- Currently not FDA approved for use as monotherapy or with insulin

- Currently not approved for use with thiazolidinediones (although approval is expected shortly)

Administration

- Twice-daily subcutaneous injection using pen device with a fixed dosage is preferred.

- Starting dosage is 5 µg before meals (breakfast and supper), increasing to 10 µg twice daily after 1 month if glucose targets are not achieved and the medication is well tolerated.

- Patients should measure blood sugar frequently, including postprandially, before starting this medication.

Side Effects

- Nausea and vomiting—usually self limited and less common on lower dosages; patients on this drug who stop eating may need to stop the medication.

- Hypoglycemia if the drug is used in combination with a sulfonylurea. The dosage of the sulfonylurea should be decreased when exenatide is started. Hypoglycemia does not occur when exenatide is used in combination with metformin alone.

- Weight loss (up to 5.5 kg [12 lb] after 2 years of treatment)

Therapeutic Benefit

- Addition of exenatide to a sulfonylurea, metformin, or both results in an absolute reduction of hemoglobin A1C value of 1 percentage point compared with placebo.

- The major effect of exenatide is the lowering of the postprandial glucose level, but a modest reduction in the fasting glucose level occurs as well.

Contraindicated in:

- Patients with gastroparesis

- Patients who are pregnant or lactating

- Children

Pramlintide (Symlin)

Pramlintide is a synthetic form of amylin, a naturally occurring peptide that is co-secreted with insulin by the beta cell. Amylin potentiates the effects of insulin. Persons with type 1 diabetes lack amylin (just as they lack insulin), and those with type 2 diabetes have reduced levels of the hormone. Like exenatide, pramlintide suppresses glucagon secretion, slows gastric emptying, and promotes satiety.

Indications

- Adjunct to insulin therapy (multiple daily injection regimens or insulin pump) in patients with type 1 or type 2 diabetes who have primarily postprandial hyperglycemia

- Can be used in patients with type 2 diabetes who use insulin, metformin, and/or a sulfonylurea

Administration

- Subcutaneous pre-meal injection is generally 60 or 120 µg in type 2 diabetes and 15, 30, 45, or 60 µg in type 1 diabetes.

- It cannot be mixed with insulin.

- Frequent blood-sugar monitoring is required, including postprandially, prior to starting pramlintide.

- Referral to an endocrinologist is usually necessary in patients considering pramlintide.

Side Effects

- Nausea and vomiting can be minimized by starting with a low dosage and increasing the dosage every 3 to 7 days, if tolerated.

- Hypoglycemia—insulin dosage should be reduced by up to 50% when starting pramlintide to minimize hypoglycemia. Patients who count carbohydrates and use rapid-acting insulin can often further decrease their risk for hypoglycemia by taking their prandial insulin after the meal, basing dosage on the actual carbohydrates consumed.

- Weight loss is usually less than 4.5 kg (10 lb).

Therapeutic Effect

- Lowers postprandial glucose level by up to 60 mg/dL when used with insulin prior to meals.

- Decreases hemoglobin A1C value by approximately 0.6%.

Contraindicated in:

- Patients with delayed gastric emptying or who are taking other drugs that delay gastric emptying

- Patients who are pregnant or lactating

- Children with diabetes

What do I need to teach my patients about other injectables?

The following information is helpful for patients taking or considering other injectables:

- *Similarities:* Both exenatide and pramlintide mimic hormones secreted along with insulin, and both help to lower postprandial glucose levels. Both must be taken by injection and have weight loss as a side effect.

- *Exenatide:* This drug mimics a hormone (GLP-1) secreted from the intestine when food enters the stomach. GLP-1 stimulates insulin secretion from the pancreas, slows down the production of glucose from the liver, and slows down the movement of food through the stomach. It is effective only for patients with type 2 diabetes whose bodies still make insulin naturally (endogenous insulin production).

- *Pramlintide:* This drug is a synthetic form of amylin, a hormone that is co-secreted with insulin from the pancreas and that lowers the postprandial glucose level. This, too, slows gastric emptying and suppresses glucagon secretion, thereby decreasing heptic glucose production. Hence, this hormone increases the effectiveness of mealtime insulin. It is effective for patients with type 1 or type 2 diabetes who take preprandial insulin injections.

- Because of the risk for hypoglycemia, frequent blood glucose monitoring is critical when these medications are initiated.

- Essential components of education for patients taking these medications include a discussion of hypoglycemia prevention, symptoms, and treatment; how to manage insulin during an acute illness; and the need for diabetes identification.

- Regarding pramlintide, discuss a plan for dosage adjustments and when to contact you or another provider about hypoglycemia, hyperglycemia, and side effects. Point out that it may take some time for the drug to work properly and that adjustments can be made to regulate the dosage of pramlintide.

Because these medications are relatively new, not all payers currently provide coverage, and many require prior authorization. Patients need to check with their insurer prior to filling the prescription.

What should I ask patients about their injected medication at each visit?

- Are you having any problems with high or low blood glucose levels?

- About how often do you miss taking this medication?

- Do you have difficulty paying for this medication?

- Are you having any problems with this medication? What specific problems have you encountered? Have you had any nausea? What have you tried to solve this problem? Did it work?

- How well do you think your treatment plan is working to manage your diabetes?

- Do you have any questions about this medication?

- How can I help most?

What facts about exenatide do patients need to know?

Some key facts to share with patients about exenatide include:

- Take exenatide twice daily, 60 minutes or less before the morning and evening meals (with meals at least 6 hours apart).

- If you miss a dose, do not take it after your meal or take a larger dosage at your next meal.

- Store both opened and unopened pens in the refrigerator. Discard the pen if it freezes or looks cloudy. Unopened vials are good until the expiration date.

- Once opened, each pen is good for 30 days. Discard after 30 days even if some medication remains.

- Opened pens can be removed from refrigeration for short periods of time. The total time pens can be unrefrigerated is a cumulative total of 6 days.

- Pen needles need to be purchased separately.

- Exenatide can be injected subcutaneously in the arm, abdomen, or thigh.

- Do not adjust the dosage based on meal size or activity level.

- Because this medication can affect the absorption of some oral medications, tell all of your health care providers that you are taking this medication.

What facts about pramlintide do patients need to know?

The following information about pramlintide should likewise be shared with patients:

- Take pramlintide right before any meal that contains at least 250 calories or 30 g of carbohydrates.

- If you miss a dose, do not take it after your meal or take a larger dosage at your next meal.

- Do not mix pramlintide in the same syringe as insulin.

- Pramlintide can be injected subcutaneously in the arm, abdomen, or thigh. It should be injected at least 2 inches from the site of your most recent insulin injection.

- Each opened vial of pramlintide is good for 28 days when stored at room temperature. Discard after 28 days even if some medication remains. Discard if the vial has been frozen or heated above room temperature (25 °C [77 °F]).

Injectable Drug Supplies

This section briefly describes some of the supplies patients on insulin or other injectable drugs need for managing their diabetes. A certified diabetes educator or other diabetes health care provider is an excellent resource for information about currently available diabetes supplies.

Syringes

Syringes are available in 0.3-cc, 0.5-cc, and 1.0-cc sizes. When initially prescribing insulin syringes, consider the potential maximum dosage per injection to insure the patient has syringes that will be able to accommodate any dosage increases that may occur following diagnosis.

The length and gauge of the syringe needle can affect comfort and absorption. The "short" (5/16-inch) needles are commonly prescribed because healthcare providers and patients perceive these as causing less discomfort than half-inch needles. However, short needles, if prescribed improperly, can be associated with more discomfort because the insulin may be delivered intradermally, rather than subcutaneously. Increased leakage is possible, contributing to variable delivery and glucose fluctuations.

Pen Injectors

Many of the injectable diabetes medications can be administered using injector devices (pens). Pens offer a greater degree of accuracy than syringes, particularly for patients with vision or dexterity problems, and are often considered more convenient than traditional syringes. However, this convenience does come at a price. Pens are often more expensive and associated with a higher copayment if a vial form of the medication is also available. Additionally, not all insurance providers cover pens, and some restrict the types of pen covered.

Some insulin pens are disposable, whereas others use disposable cartridges. All pens use specially designed pen needles. As with syringes, the pen needles are available in various lengths and diameters. Just as with syringe use, initial patient instruction with ongoing evaluation of technique is critical to avoid errors in medication delivery.

The American Diabetes Association's annual Resource Guide (www.diabetes.org/diabetes-forecast/resource-guide.jsp) provides an up-to-date listing and description of the pens available.

Glucagon

All patients with type 1 diabetes should be provided with a prescription for a glucagon emergency kit to be used for treatment of severe hypoglycemia. A family member or caregiver must be instructed in how and when to administer glucagon, which is reserved for when the patient cannot safely take anything orally to treat a severe hypoglycemic event or reaction. Patients with type 2 diabetes who are on insulin and have a history of severe hypoglycemia may also benefit from having a glucagon emergency kit available. Because such kits are expensive and not always covered by insurance, the decision to prescribe one for patients with type 2 diabetes should be based on the individual clinical situation.

Because glucagon is used infrequently, if at all, by most patients, it is likely to reach its expiration date. The need for a new prescription can be part of the routine assessment of patients with diabetes.

Ketone Test Strips

Ketone monitoring is used to assess insulin deficiency in type 1 diabetes during hyperglycemia, acute illness, or stress. In patients with type 2 diabetes, regular ketone monitoring is not recommended, except during pregnancy. At least one blood glucose meter is also able to measure blood ketones. Ketone monitoring is an essential component of sick-day management for patients with type 1 diabetes. In addition, patients with type 1 diabetes who are using insulin pump therapy should monitor their ketones to assess insulin delivery, especially during unexplained hyperglycemia.

Beta Cell Replacement Therapies

Beta cell replacement therapy, which offers an intuitive method to obtain normoglycemia, attracts inquiry from patients and providers alike. Currently, beta cell replacement is reserved for those who have lost significant secretory capacity, usually because of autoimmune diabetes, pancreatitis, or pancreatic surgery. Available options for beta cell replacement include whole-organ pancreas transplantation and islet transplantation.

Whole-organ pancreas transplantation is generally considered an acceptable alternative to continued exogenous insulin in patients with diabetes who have imminent or established end-stage kidney disease and have had or plan to have a kidney transplant. The procedure involves transplanting a donor pancreas into the peritoneal cavity with drainage of the digestive juices of the exocrine pancreas into the ileum (or, less commonly, the bladder) and drainage of the

insulin-containing venous return into the portal or systemic circulation. Quality of life studies show improvement after pancreas transplantation, often with normalization of A1C values and stabilization or improvement in many complications of diabetes. One-year graft survival rates are 85% for simultaneous pancreas-kidney transplants, 78% for pancreas transplants after kidney transplantation, and 77% for pancreas transplants alone; 5-year graft survival rates are 69%, 46%, and 42%, respectively. Because graft survival rates are far superior with simultaneous kidney-pancreas transplantation, such surgery is the preferred method.

Pancreas transplantation has significant morbidity and carries a small, but not negligible, risk of mortality. Potential complications include intra-abdominal infection and abscess, vascular graft thromboses, and anastomotic leakage. Cytomegalovirus infection, cytopenia, malignancy, hypertension, hyperlipidemia, insulin resistance, and other metabolic abnormalities have also all been seen secondary to the required immunosuppression after transplantation.

With islet transplantation, the endocrine portions of the pancreas—the islets of Langerhans—are transplanted, usually via an infusion of isolated islets into the portal vein of the liver. Many insurers will at least partially cover the autotransplantation of islets in persons undergoing pancreatectomy for pancreatitis. In patients with pancreatitis who have not had prior pancreatic surgery, insulin-independence rates after autotransplantation may exceed 70%. An added benefit is that immunosuppression is not required, as in allotransplantation. In contrast, islet allotransplantation, which is currently being studied for the treatment of type 1 diabetes, remains an experimental procedure and is not covered by insurance. Medicare may pay some of the costs associated with participation in a National Institutes of Health–sponsored clinical trial. In most clinical trials, islet allotransplantation candidates have been relatively thin and insulin sensitive, minimizing the number of islets required for transplantation.

Complications related to islet transplantation have included peritoneal hemorrhage, portal vein thrombosis, peri-islet hepatic steatosis, and transient transaminitis. In addition, oral ulcerations, diarrhea, weight loss, decline in glomerular filtration rate, proteinuria, cytopenia, hypertension, hyperlipidemia, pneumonitis, and small bowel ulcerations have all been associated with the requisite immunosuppression for allotransplantation. The most frequent indication for islet allotransplantation has been severe, life-threatening hypoglycemia. Although hypoglycemia is much improved after islet transplantation, the glycemia achieved remains inferior to that seen with whole-organ transplants. Insulin independence in those with type 1 diabetes has also been fleeting. The median duration of insulin independence is only 15 months, and fewer than 10% of recipients remain insulin independent at 5 years.

9. Obesity

Obesity significantly increases the risk of developing type 2 diabetes, and the health consequences of obesity are more severe among patients with diabetes. In particular, central obesity is independently associated with insulin resistance and increased cardiovascular risk.

Classification of Obesity

Body mass index (BMI) is used to classify obesity (**Table 9-1**). BMI is calculated by dividing a patient's weight in kilograms by the square of the height in meters (kg/m^2). The BMI can be misleading in very muscular persons, who may have a high BMI but will not necessarily be obese, and those who have lost significant muscle mass, who may have a low BMI but are obese. A chart for calculating and interpreting BMI is included (*Body Mass Index Table*) in Chapter 9 of the *Diabetes Care Guide Toolkit*. In addition, a BMI calculator is provided on the accompanying CD-ROM and on the ACP Diabetes Portal (http://diabetes.acponline.org).

The first steps in the treatment of obesity and the cornerstones of ongoing weight management are counseling on dietary and behavioral modification (exercise) and establishing individual goals for weight loss and the management of comorbidities. According to the ACP practice guidelines for the management of obesity, pharmacotherapy may be considered if goals are not met with diet and exercise. Bariatric surgery is a treatment option for patients with a BMI >40 (morbidly obese) and with obesity-related comorbidities who have not succeeded with diet and exercise regimens. **Figure 9-1** summarizes the ACP 2005 clinical practice guidelines for management of obesity.

Helping Your Patients Lose Weight

How can I help my overweight or obese patients lose weight?

Lifestyle changes, including regular exercise and caloric reduction, are the first steps in the management of obesity and remain the foundations of therapy, even when additional treatment for obesity is begun.

- Measure the patient's BMI and waist circumference and inform him or her of the results. (Waist circumference should be measured just above the iliac crests, with the tape measure pulled snugly around waist.) Women with a waist circumference of 35 inches or more and men with a waist circumference of 40 inches or more are at higher risk of developing diabetes.

- Assess the patient's readiness to lose weight, including:

  - Reasons and motivation for weight loss;

  - Previous attempts at weight loss;

  - Support from family and friends;

  - Understanding of the risks and benefits of weight loss;

  - Attitudes toward physical activity;

  - Potential barriers to losing weight;

  - On a scale of 1 to 10, the level of importance placed on weight loss and the patient's confidence in the ability to succeed.

- Help the patient set realistic weight loss goals and specific diet and physical activity strategies (**Table 9-2**). *Setting Your Self-Management*

Table 9-1. World Health Organization Classification of Body Weight

Body Mass Index	Classification
<18.5	Underweight (thin)
18.5-24.9	Normal
25-29.9	Pre-obese (overweight)
30-34.9	Class 1 obese
35-39.9	Class 2 obese
>40	Class 3 obese (morbid obesity)

Goal and *Your Self-Management Workbook* in Chapter 2 of the *Diabetes Care Guide Toolkit* can help patients with goal setting.

• Recognize that to successfully lose weight, patients need ongoing support and follow-up. Offer referral to a registered dietitian and have a list of local weight loss programs and support services when referring patients seeking to lose weight.

The National Institutes of Health's *Practical Guide to Identification and Treatment of Overweight and Obesity in Adults* provides a step-by-step guide to the management of overweight and obese patients, including an appendix of patient handouts and self-management tools related to diet, physical activity, and behavioral modification. This full guide is available at `www.nhlbi.nih.gov/guidelines/obesity/prctgd_b.pdf`.

How can I help my patients incorporate more exercise into their lives?

Exercise does not have to be strenuous to provide benefits. Patients of all ages can benefit by gradually incorporating more physical activity into their lives—even a little bit of physical activity is better than none. Ask your patients who do not currently engage in regular exercise to think of one thing they are interested in and willing to do to begin to incorporate a few minutes of increased physical activity into each day. For example, as part of a short-term, specific action plan, patients can try to walk 10 minutes after lunch three times a week. Help patients identify the activities that they would like to try and that fit into their lives. Patients may

not realize that even ordinary tasks, such as gardening, playing with grandchildren, and housework, entail moderate physical activity. They may not realize that recreational activities, such as dancing or golf, are excellent ways of getting exercise.

In addition, goals must be realistic. Reaching a targeted, realistic goal will increase patients' self-confidence and may enable them to gradually build up to more minutes of physical activity and more intensive physical activity.

The Centers for Disease Control and Prevention currently recommends the following targets:

• Moderate-intensity physical activities: ≥30 minutes on 5 or more days each week *or*

• Vigorous-intensity physical activity: ≥20 minutes on 3 or more days each week

Additionally, many experts recommend that persons with diabetes who are planning to begin a vigorous exercise program (more intense than brisk walking) should first undergo cardiac stress testing, although no definitive evidence supports this recommendation.

Dietary Interventions

To achieve weight loss, quantitative caloric reduction must accompany qualitative changes in food intake. The Joslin Diabetes Center has developed evidence-based guidelines for weight reduction in obese and overweight patients with diabetes. These include:

1. Structured lifestyle plan that combines dietary modification and exercise;

2. Modest and gradual weight reduction (0.5 kg [1 lb] every 1–2 weeks);

3. Daily caloric reduction of 250–500 calories, with total caloric intake not less than 1000–1200 calories/day for women and 1200–1600 calories/day for men;

4. Individualized weight reduction program to achieve target BMI (18.5–25.0 or agreed-upon goal);

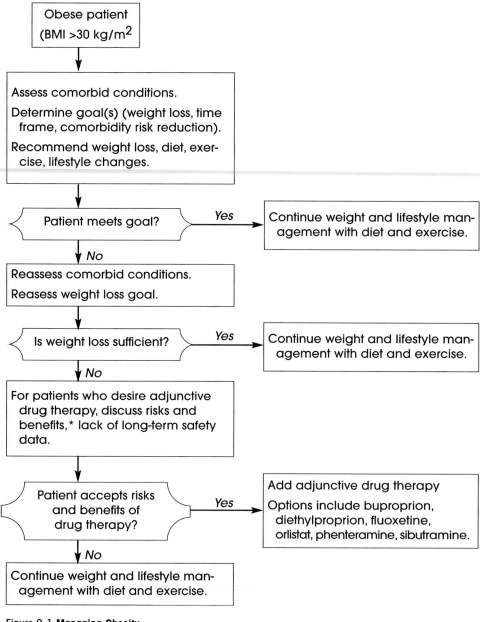

Figure 9-1 **Managing Obesity**

BMI = body mass index. *Assess side effects and efficacy; no data are available past 12 months except for orlistat.

Adapted with permission from Snow V, Barry P, Fitterman N, Qaseem A, Weiss K. Pharmacologic and surgical management of obesity in primary care: a clinical practice guideline from the American College of Physicians. Ann Intern Med. 2005;142:526.

diet. **Table 9-3** summarizes these dietary composition recommendations.

All patients with diabetes (particularly those on insulin or insulin secretagogues) who plan to make significant quantitative or qualitative changes in their diet must discuss these changes with their physician to reduce the risk of hypoglycemia. Blood glucose records need to be monitored weekly, and blood pressure and lipid levels need to be followed regularly.

Liquid meal replacements marketed to persons with diabetes are available over the counter, including Boost Glycemic Control, Boost Diabetic, Sugar Free Slimfast, and Glucerna. Patients use them with or without the advice of a physician. Very-low-calorie diets (<800 calories/day, available commercially as powders) should only be used if patients are under the close supervision of a physician. Low-calorie diets in combination with regular physical activity should be attempted before initiating a very-low-calorie diet. These diets are contraindicated in patients with cardiovascular, renal, or hepatic disease; type 1 diabetes; protein-wasting diseases; and cancer. Persons with psychiatric disease or a history of an eating disorder should also not follow a very-low-calorie diet.

5. Regular follow-up with a registered dietitian to learn and practice portion control.

In addition, the Joslin guidelines advise replacing refined carbohydrates and processed grains with low–glycemic index foods, avoiding severe carbohydrate restriction, limiting saturated fat intake, and including adequate protein in the

Table 9-2. Recommended Options for Weight Loss

Caloric Intake

Moderate decreases in caloric intake (e.g., 500–1000 calories/day) will result in slow but progressive weight loss.
Diets low in fat (~30% of calories) and saturated fat (<10% of calories) are recommended to reduce cardiovascular risk in obese patients.
Dietary guidance should be individualized and allow for patient food preferences and approaches to reduce caloric intake.
Very-low-calorie diets (<800 calories/day) are only recommended with appropriate medical supervision and monitoring.
Reducing portion sizes, selecting low-calorie foods, and using cooking methods that reduce fat intake can decrease overall caloric intake.

Physical Activity

Developing a regular pattern of exercise is central to successful long-term weight loss.
Lifestyle physical activity can be effective in producing weight loss, changing body composition, and improving risk factors for cardiovascular disease.
30–45 minutes of moderate-level physical activity is recommended 3–5 days per week initially. (Gradually, duration and frequency should increase.)
Physical activity does not need to occur in a single session to be beneficial.
Exercise programs should be determined by patient preferences, experience, physical abilities, and access to facilities.

Behavior Modification

Self-monitoring: Observe and record target behaviors.
Stimulus control and stress management: Identify and modify cues that promote overeating or inactivity. Manage stress that can trigger overeating and lead to relapse.
Rewards: Identify desirable and timely rewards that reinforce achievement of specific goals.
Cognitive restructuring: Increase awareness of internal dialogue and negative perceptions of self; develop positive "self-talk."
Social support: Include others in weight loss plans to provide encouragement.

Adapted with permission from: Pi-Sunyer FX, Daly AE, Funnell MM, Heber D, Kushner R, Rubin RR, et al, eds. Clinical Management of Obesity: With Special Attention to Type 2 Diabetes. Alexandria, Va.: American Diabetes Association; 2004. Copyright © 2004 American Diabetes Association.

How can I help my patients develop healthier eating habits?

As with physical activity, ask your patients to think of one thing they are interested in and willing to do to improve their eating habits (for example, eating one additional vegetable serving a day). Discuss the nutritional guidelines below with your patients.

• Eat more fruits and vegetables, legumes, and whole and minimally processed grains. Carbohydrates should make up about 25% of daily caloric intake.

• The "plate method" is a convenient way for some patients to monitor the amounts and proportions of carbohydrates, proteins, and nonstarchy vegetables in their diets. (See Chapter 5, Helping Patients Make Lifestyle Changes.) In addition, *Rate Your Plate* in Chapter 5 of the *Diabetes Care Guide Toolkit* is a handout that patients can use to quickly assess the nutritional value of their meals.

• Limit refined carbohydrates such as pasta, white bread, and low-fiber cereal. (A minimum of 20–35 grams of fiber per day is recommended.)

• Eat mono- and polyunsaturated fats (e.g., olive oil, canola oil, nuts/seeds, and fish, particularly those high in omega-3 fatty acids). Oily fish twice per week, such as salmon, herring, lake trout, sardines, and albacore tuna, is an ample source of omega-3 fatty acids.

• Foods high in dietary cholesterol, such as egg yolks, red meat, whole-fat dairy foods, and organ meats, should be limited.

Which patients are candidates for weight loss pharmacotherapy or surgery?

Pharmacologic Approaches to Weight Loss

If a trial of diet and exercise is not successful, pharmacotherapy may be appropriate. The U.S. Food and Drug Administration and the National Heart, Lung, and Blood Institute both consider

Table 9-3. Dietary Composition Recommendations for Obese or Overweight Adults with Type 2 Diabetes*

Dietary Component	% of Caloric Intake	Daily Intake	Notes
Carbohydrates	~40%	Not less than 130 g daily	Low-glycemic index foods (oats, barley, whole grains, fruits, legumes) should replace refined carbohydrates (potatoes, white bread).
Fiber		25–30 g daily initially; if tolerated, up to 50 g daily	Preferably from fruits and vegetables. Fiber supplements if needed.
Fat Saturated Polyunsaturated Monounsaturated	~30%–35% <10%† 10% 15%–20%		Mono- and polyunsaturated fats include olive and canola oil, nuts/seeds, oily fish (salmon, herring, trout, sardines, fresh tuna).Saturated fats are found in pork, beef, lamb, high-fat dairy products.Fast food and commercially baked foods are high in trans fats and should be avoided.
Cholesterol		<300 mg daily†	Limit egg yolks, red meat, whole fat dairy foods, shellfish.
Protein	20%–30%‡		Protein should come from lean meats, low-fat dairy products, or tofu/tempeh/seitan products rather than from high-saturated fat animal sources. Protein is associated with increased satiety and can help maintain lean body mass during weight reduction.

Adapted with permission from: Joslin Diabetes Center. Clinical nutrition guideline for overweight and obese adults with type 2 diabetes, prediabetes, or who are at high risk for developing type 2 diabetes. Copyright © 2005. Available at: www.joslin.org/managing_your_diabetes_joslin_clinical_guidelines.asp. Accessed 3 October 2006.

*Any meal plan modifications should first be discussed with a registered dietitian (RD) or a qualified health-care provider. The diet composition, described above, is for general guidance only and may be individualized by the RD or health-care provider according to clinical judgment.

†In persons with an LDL cholesterol level >100 mg/dL, saturated fat should be <7% of total daily caloric intake and cholesterol intake should be <200 mg/day.

‡Persons with a glomerular filtration rate <60 mL/min should consult with a nephrologist before increasing protein in their diet.

pharmacotherapy appropriate for persons with a BMI >27 who have significant comorbidities—including diabetes, hypertension, and dyslipidemia—and those with a BMI >30 regardless of comorbidities. A 6-month trial of diet and exercise should be attempted first. Medications approved for the treatment of obesity work by suppressing appetite or inhibiting lipase. Several medications used for weight loss are listed in **Table 9-4**. Only sibutramine and orlistat are approved for long-term use. The patient and physician must discuss medication side effects and safety data, as well as the fact that weight loss achieved through pharmacotherapy is often not sustained.

Contraindications to pharmacotherapy for obesity are as follows:

• Pregnancy or lactation (pregnancy test should be done before prescribing)

• Unstable cardiac disease

• Uncontrolled hypertension (systolic blood pressure >180 mm Hg or diastolic blood pressure >110 mm Hg)

• Severe systemic illness (e.g., cancer)

• Psychiatric illness

• History of an eating disorder

• Concomitant use of monoamine oxidase inhibitors, migraine medications, or other adrenergic medications

Surgical Approaches to Weight Loss

The National Heart, Lung, and Blood Institute considers bariatric surgery an option for persons with a BMI >40 and no comorbidities or a BMI

Table 9-4. Medications Used for Weight Loss

Drug	Mechanism of Action	Side Effects
Sibutramine*†	Appetite suppressant: combined norepinephrine and serotonin reuptake inhibitor	Modest increases in heart rate and blood pressure, nervousness, insomnia
Phentermine*†	Appetite suppressant: sympathomimetic amine	Cardiovascular, gastrointestinal
Diethylpropion*†	Appetite suppressant: sympathomimetic amine	Palpitations, tachycardia, insomnia, gastrointestinal
Orlistat*	Lipase inhibitor: decreased absorption of fat	Diarrhea, flatulence, bloating, abdominal pain, dyspepsia
Bupropion	Appetite suppressant: mechanism unknown	Paresthesia, insomnia, central nervous system effects
Fluoxetine	Appetite suppressant: selective serotonin reuptake inhibitor	Agitation, nervousness, gastrointestinal
Sertraline	Appetite suppressant: selective serotonin reuptake inhibitor	Agitation, nervousness, gastrointestinal
Topiramate	Mechanism unknown	Paresthesia, changes in taste
Zonisamide	Mechanism unknown	Somnolence, dizziness, nausea

*Approved by the U.S. Food and Drug Administration for weight loss.

†Drug Enforcement Administration schedule IV.

Reprinted with permission from: Snow V, Barry P, Fitterman N, Qaseem A, Weiss K. Pharmacologic and surgical management of obesity in primary care: a clinical practice guideline from the American College of Physicians. Ann Intern Med. 2005;142:525-31.

of >35 with comorbidities. The ACP guidelines for bariatric surgery are somewhat narrower— BMI >40 with comorbidities. A patient being considered for bariatric surgery should have already tried diet and exercise. Patients must go through a rigorous screening process, including an assessment of social supports and willingness and ability to adhere to close medical follow-up. A discussion of the long-term side effects of surgery, including gallbladder disease, malabsorption, and the possible need for reoperation, must occur before surgical intervention. If surgery is planned, the ACP recommends referral to high-volume centers with surgeons experienced in bariatric surgery.

Surgical treatments of obesity include restrictive procedures (adjustable gastric banding or vertical banded gastroplasty) and procedures that produce malabsorption (Roux-en-Y gastric bypass, biliopancreatic bypass).

No randomized, controlled trials comparing surgical and medical management of morbid obesity are available. A large Swedish observational study followed patients who underwent bariatric surgery and compared them with a weight-matched cohort that followed medical management. Surgically treated patients experienced sustained weight loss compared with medically treated counterparts. Because the surgically treated patients were self-selected, surgery cannot be viewed as superior to medical management for all patients. The incidence of hypertension, diabetes, and dyslipidemia were improved after 2 years in patients who underwent surgery, but not all of these improvements were sustained at 10 years.

Contraindications to surgery include psychiatric illness and substance abuse. Perioperative complications of surgery occur in approximately 10% of patients and include infection, leaks at the anastamosis site, and pulmonary embolus. As many as 25% of patients develop nutritional deficiencies, some of which are not reversible if discovered late. Patients must take vitamin and mineral supplements indefinitely following gastric surgery.

10. Hyperlipidemia and Hypertension

Patients with diabetes have accelerated atherosclerosis and an increased incidence of premature cardiovascular events. Epidemiologic studies and major clinical trials have shown that cardiovascular risk factors—including hypercholesterolemia, hypertension, and cigarette smoking—have an increased impact on the incidence and progression of cardiovascular events. These risk factors often coexist as key components of the metabolic syndrome. In particular, patients with type 2 diabetes have an increased prevalence of lipid abnormalities (>80%, based on current goals) and hypertension (>60%). Moreover, patients with type 1 diabetes that is accompanied by renal disease and those with type 2 diabetes that is poorly controlled have additional lipid abnormalities, including high triglyceride levels and low HDL cholesterol levels.

Because of the markedly increased risk of cardiovascular disease in patients with diabetes and the established evidence for improved outcome with optimal management, various clinical practice guidelines (of the American College of Physicians [ACP], the American Diabetes Association, the American Heart Association, and others), advocate stricter goals for such patients than for those without diabetes. According to available recent national statistics, however, the control of glycemia, blood pressure, and LDL cholesterol is not being achieved in most patients with diabetes.

Hyperlipidemia

Patients with diabetes are at high risk for cardiovascular disease, even in the absence of established coronary artery disease (CAD). Multiple studies have shown that lipid-lowering therapy in patients with type 2 diabetes leads to a 22% to 24% reduction in major cardiovascular events. The class of drugs whose use is supported by the best evidence is statins.

Although advisory bodies agree on the benefit of statins in reducing cardiovascular risk in diabetes, specific recommendations vary. For example, the National Cholesterol Education Program Adult Treatment Panel III (ATP III) recommends a goal of less than 100 mg/dL for the LDL cholesterol level in patients with diabetes. For patients with diabetes and CAD, ATP III recommends an even lower target of <70 mg/dL. Evidence from the Heart Protection Study and Collaborative Diabetes Atorvastatin Study (CARDS) supports the use of statins in patients with diabetes and CAD regardless of the baseline LDL cholesterol level. Similarly, ACP recommends that persons with diabetes take at least moderate dosages of statins but does not specify LDL cholesterol targets.

Combination therapy using a statin with either a fibrate or niacin to lower the level of triglycerides or raise the level of HDL cholesterol may be considered in high-risk patients, including those with CAD or multiple risk factors, but evidence regarding the risks and benefits of such an approach is lacking until the completion of ongoing clinical trials.

Statins and fibrates are contraindicated during pregnancy and lactation.

What are the lipid goals for patients with diabetes?

Although consensus has not been reached, the following lipid goals are reasonable for patients with diabetes:

- Lipid goals for adults with diabetes and no additional cardiovascular risk factors:

  - LDL cholesterol level <100 mg/dL

  - Triglyceride level <150 mg/dL

  - HDL cholesterol level >40 mg/dL in men and >50 mg/dL in women

- In patients age 40 years or older who have diabetes but no cardiovascular disease, consider pharmacologic therapy, preferably with a statin, to achieve an LDL cholesterol goal of <100 mg/dL. In patients younger than 40 years who have diabetes but no cardiovascular disease, consider pharmacologic therapy to achieve this goal if additional risk factors are present.

- In patients with diabetes and cardiovascular disease, consider pharmacologic treatment to achieve an LDL cholesterol goal of <70 mg/dL, regardless of age.

- Test annually, or more often if needed to achieve lipid goals.

Lifestyle interventions to reduce lipid levels include reducing saturated fat and cholesterol intake, smoking cessation, weight loss (if indicated), and increased physical activity. Suggestions for helping patients make such changes are discussed in Chapter 5 (Helping Patients Make Lifestyle Changes) and Chapter 12 (Complications of Diabetes).

What do I need to teach patients about lipid management and diabetes?

- Stress the link between diabetes and heart disease. Although heart disease is the leading cause of death for people with diabetes, most patients do not recognize this as a complication of diabetes.

- Stress the importance of blood glucose management along with lipid management as a strategy to prevent heart disease.

- Provide information about lipid goals for people with diabetes and explain the importance of HDL cholesterol (levels should be high), LDL cholesterol (levels should be low), and triglyceride levels, along with specific strategies to improve each reading.

- Refer to a dietitian for dietary and exercise counseling.

- If lipid-lowering medications are prescribed, provide written information about the name, dosage, timing, and side effects, as well as when to take for maximum effectiveness.

- Because of financial or other concerns, many patients choose to take one of their medications but not others. Stress the action and synergistic nature of multiple medications.

- Ask that patients contact you about side effects rather than stopping the medication.

- Provide instructions on how to handle forgotten and missed doses.

Hypertension

Improved blood pressure control in patients with diabetes markedly reduces cardiovascular events and overall mortality. The occurrence of microvascular complications, including retinopathy and renal disease, is reduced when blood pressure control is improved.

What are the blood pressure goals for patients with diabetes?

As with lipid management, organizations agree on the importance of treating hypertension in patients with diabetes, but they have minor differences in their specific recommendations. The ACP advocates a target blood pressure of no more than 135/80 mm Hg for persons with diabetes, whereas the 7th Joint National Committee on Prevention, Detection, Evaluation, and Treatment of High Blood Pressure (JNC-7) recommends a target blood pressure of 130/80 mm Hg for such persons.

The JNC-7 emphasizes the importance of systolic blood pressure as a cardiovascular risk factor, particularly in persons older than 50 years. However, the optimal systolic blood pressure target in patients with hypertension and diabetes is not known with certainty. The United Kingdom Prospective Diabetes Study (UKPDS) showed that lower risk occurs with a systolic blood pressure below 120 mm Hg, although no actual threshold was observed for any endpoint. For each 10 mm Hg decrease in systolic pressure, the study found a 12% reduction for any complications related to diabetes.

The minor differences in blood pressure target recommendations should be considered in the context of the fact that only 31% of persons in the United States with hypertension and diabetes have a blood pressure lower than 140/90 mm Hg.

- Blood pressure should be measured at each visit.

- Patients with diabetes often develop autonomic insufficiency. In patients with signs of end-organ damage and in those reporting dizziness, orthostatic blood pressure measurements should be monitored.

How do I treat hypertension in my patients with diabetes?

Lifestyle Interventions

In patients with systolic pressures of 130 to 139 mm Hg and diastolic pressures of 80 to 89 mm Hg, lifestyle and behavioral therapy may be attempted for 3 months, although some authorities believe the risk of hypertension in diabetes is so great that pharmacologic therapy should be instituted initially along with lifestyle modifications. (See Chapter 5, Helping Patients Make Lifestyle Changes.) Weight loss, salt restriction, and exercise are all important. The National Heart, Lung, and Blood Institute developed an excellent, effective diet known as the *Dietary Approaches to Stop Hypertension (DASH)* eating plan. If goals are not met, pharmacologic treatment should be instituted.

Pharmacologic Treatment

The Antihypertensive and Lipid-Lowering Treatment to Prevent Heart Attack Trial (ALLHAT) found that high-risk patients, including patients with diabetes, have better cardiovascular outcomes when started on thiazide monotherapy rather than on an angiotensin-converting enzyme (ACE) inhibitor. However, nearly all patients with diabetes and hypertension will require the addition of an ACE inhibitor and an angiotensin II receptor blocker (ARB) to attain blood pressure goals.

ACE inhibitors and ARBs have been shown to provide renal protective benefits in diabetes. The ACP suggests a thiazide diuretic or an ACE inhibitor as a first-line agent for blood pressure control in patients with diabetes. ACE inhibitors and ARBs are contraindicated during pregnancy.

Consider referral to a nephrologist if any of the following are present:

- Lack of blood pressure control, despite multiple drugs

- A progressive decline in glomerular filtration rate

- Marked hyperkalemia

What do I need to teach patients about blood pressure management and diabetes?

Some steps to help patients with diabetes manage their blood pressure include:

- Stress the links between diabetes and hypertension, cardiovascular disease, and stroke.

- Stress the importance of blood pressure management and blood glucose management as strategies to prevent both the microvascular and macrovascular complications of diabetes.

- Provide information about blood pressure goals for people with diabetes and the importance of both systolic and diastolic readings.

- Refer to a dietitian for dietary and exercise counseling.

- If antihypertensive medications are prescribed, provide written information about the name, dosage, timing, and side effects, as well as when to take the drugs for maximum effectiveness.

- Because of financial or other concerns, many patients choose to take one of their medications but not others. Stress the action and synergistic nature of multiple medications.

- Ask that patients contact you about side effects rather than stopping the medication.

- Provide instructions on how to handle forgotten and missed doses.

What should I ask patients about their lipid and hypertension medications at each visit?

Monitoring patients' compliance with their lipid and antihypertensive therapy should be part of each visit. Suggested questions to ask follow:

- Are you having any side effects? (Ask men specifically about erectile dysfunction as a side effect of antihypertensive agents.)

- Are you having trouble paying for any of your medications?

- About how often do you miss taking your medications?

- Are you taking any vitamins or herbal or natural products?

- Do you have difficulty taking your medications? What specific problems have you encountered? What have you tried to solve this problem? What other options do you think may be effective?

- How well do you think your treatment plan is working to manage your cholesterol levels and blood pressure?

- Do you have any questions about your medications?

- How can I help most?

A handout that patients can use to record their test results and dates—along with their individualized treatment goals—is provided in Chapter 10 of the *Diabetes Care Guide Toolkit (Your Diabetes Test Record)*. Because this form contains personal medical information, patients must consciously decide who will have access to it. Also in the toolkit, *The ABCs to Good Diabetes Self-Care* lists the recommended frequency of essential examinations, immunizations, and medications. This tool includes a place to record self-management goals that you can discuss with the patient.

11. Depression and Cognitive Dysfunction

Depression

Depression is approximately twice as common in patients with diabetes (ranging from 15% to 30%) than in the general population. The odds of major depression is increased in patients with diabetes who also have two or more coexisting chronic conditions, such as hypertension, coronary artery disease, or arthritis. Diabetes and depression increase the risk of death from all causes of mortality.

The effect that treatment of depression has on glycemic control is not well defined in these patients. However, the presence of depression may play an important role by affecting a patient's ability to adapt and manage his or her disease (e.g., take medications, exercise, and make dietary modifications).

How do I screen my patients for depression?

We need to be aware of the high prevalence of depression among patients with diabetes and proactively screen for depression. Various tools are used to screen patients for depression, but evidence favoring any particular tool is lacking. The U.S. Preventive Services Task Force suggests the "two simple questions" approach:

- "Over the past 2 weeks, have you felt down, depressed, or hopeless?"

- "Over the past 2 weeks, have you felt little interest or pleasure in doing things?"

If the patient answers yes to either of these questions, consider asking the follow-up question, "Is this something for which you would like help?" A positive screen should prompt additional questioning to establish a diagnosis and initiate a plan for treatment and follow-up.

What do patients with diabetes need to know about depression?

- Stress that depression is common and is not a sign of weakness or personal failure.

- Inform patients that depression is treatable with medication and/or therapy, although combining both is usually more effective.

- If medications are prescribed, provide specific information about their dosage, timing, and any side effects. Point out that the medications require time to take effect and that if one medication does not help, others can be used.

- Provide information about community resources for low-cost or free mental health resources.

- Even if clinical depression is not present, remind patients that negative emotions (anger, guilt, frustration, sadness) are common among people with diabetes, both initially and throughout their lives. Ask that they let you know if they believe they are depressed or would benefit from counseling.

Cognitive Dysfunction

Cognitive dysfunction has been associated with both type 1 and type 2 diabetes, with a 1.5-fold greater risk of cognitive decline and a 1.6-fold increase in risk of future dementia. In older patients with type 2 diabetes, the risk of Alzheimer's disease is increased.

In type 1 diabetes, impairment in learning and memory, problem solving, and mental and motor speed has been observed. In type 2 diabetes, cognitive dysfunction is seen more consistently in areas of attention and concentration, verbal memory, visuospatial memory, language, and psychomotor speed.

Cognitive dysfunction can make it difficult for patients with diabetes to follow medical, nutritional, and exercise regimens, which increases the risk of treatment complications: for example, omission of meals, leading to hypoglycemia, or incorrect dosage or timing of insulin injections or oral medications. Patients or their caregivers may not recognize the complications of medical therapy—especially hypoglycemia—and may underreport them to you and other providers. In patients with cognitive dysfunction, the treatment regimen should be simplified so that the patient is able to follow the recommendations safely. In addition, the goal for glycemic control should be adjusted to achieve the best control possible, given the patient's ability to comply, without the risk of hypoglycemia.

If a patient is suspected of having cognitive dysfunction, referral to a mental health care provider is recommended for a definite diagnosis. In addition, provide diabetes education to family members or other caregivers of a patient with cognitive dysfunction to ensure the safety of the patient. Assessing a caregiver's ability to manage diabetes is important, particularly if the caregiver is elderly or also has health issues. In addition, referral for home health care or to other community resources may be needed.

Which patients with diabetes should be screened for cognitive dysfunction?

Cognitive dysfunction should be considered in all patients with diabetes. In many patients, cognitive dysfunction can be subtle, especially in early stages, and remain undiagnosed. Patients who make repeated errors in medication intake or judgment, who fail to achieve better glycemic control after reasonable efforts, or who seem overwhelmed by disease management should be suspected of having cognitive dysfunction. Many experts recommend screening for cognitive dysfunction in all elderly patients with diabetes because of its higher prevalence in this population and the risks of treatment complications. Tests such as the clock-drawing test and the Mini–Mental State Examination can be quickly administered in a primary care office to screen for cognitive dysfunction.

12. Complications of Diabetes

Risks for Complications in Diabetes

Persons with diabetes are at increased risk for macrovascular disease; microvascular disease, including retinopathy and nephropathy; peripheral and autonomic neuropathies; and lower extremity disease.

- Diabetic retinopathy is the leading cause of noncongenital blindness among adults.

- Diabetes is the most common cause of end-stage kidney disease in the United States, especially among Native American, Hispanic, and African American persons. One quarter to one third of patients with type 1 or type 2 diabetes develop some degree of nephropathy.

- Diabetes doubles the risk for cardiovascular disease in men and triples it in women (data from the Multiple Risk Factor Intervention Trial [MRFIT]).

- Patients with diabetes are several-fold more likely to have peripheral arterial disease than patients without diabetes.

- Peripheral arterial disease and foot ulcers in patients with diabetes account for two thirds of all nontraumatic amputations performed in the United States.

Screening for and prevention of these complications are fundamental to the care of patients with diabetes and are important components of quality of care initiatives for diabetes.

When does screening for complications need to begin for patients with a diagnosis of diabetes?

For type 2 diabetes, screening for complications should be initiated at the time of diagnosis because the disease may have been present for several years prior to actual diagnosis. Indeed, postprandial hyperglycemia, as caused by impaired glucose tolerance, is by itself a risk factor for the development of cardiovascular disease. Screening for complications should generally begin 1 year after diagnosis in patients with type 1 diabetes because that is when rates of complications (such as retinopathy) begin to rise.

Preventing Complications

Improved blood pressure control substantially reduces the risks of cardiovascular events and death. In addition, for any abnormal serum cholesterol level, patients with diabetes have more coronary disease than do patients without diabetes, so lipid control along with blood pressure control is especially important in this population. Lipid control and blood pressure control are discussed in greater detail in Chapter 10 (Hyperlipidemia and Hypertension).

Maintaining excellent glycemic and blood pressure control is essential to protect against the development of progressive nephropathy and retinopathy. In the Epidemiology of Diabetes Intervention and Complications (EDIC) study, the benefits of intensive glycemic control in reducing the risk of microvascular complications continued after 7 years of follow-up, despite the convergence of hemoglobin A1C values in the intensively and the conventionally managed groups.

Lifestyle Modifications

Weight reduction (in the presence of obesity), exercise, and a low-calorie, low-fat, high–complex carbohydrate diet are all important in preventing or delaying diabetes-related cardiovascular complications. In several trials, exercise has been found to improve cardiovascular outcomes and glycemic control among patients with type 2 diabetes. A meta-analysis of controlled trials that examined the effect of exercise on patients with type 2 diabetes found that exercise training reduced hemoglobin A1C values by 0.7 percentage point. A recent study estimated that one death per year would be prevented for every 61 adults with diabetes who walked at least 2 hours per week. Suggestions for helping your patients lose weight and exercise are discussed in Chapter 5 (Helping Patients Make Lifestyle Changes).

Further, another meta-analysis of cardiovascular risk reduction trials showed that cessation of smoking had a much greater benefit on survival than most other interventions. Helping patients who smoke to stop smoking is thus one of the most important aspects of prevention for smokers. In some studies, smoking has also been associated with increased progression of retinopathy and peripheral neuropathy.

How do I discuss smoking cessation with my patients who smoke?

- Ask: "Is smoking a problem for you? Are you interested in quitting?"

- Although patients indicate they know that smoking is generally harmful, they rarely know how it specifically relates to them. A comment such as the following may be helpful: "I am especially concerned about your smoking because you have diabetes, and this greatly increases your risk for other medical complications."

- Offer smoking cessation strategies, such as referrals to smoking cessation programs, medications that help with smoking cessation, and nicotine replacement products.

Pharmaceutical Measures

Microvascular Disease

- For patients who have microalbuminuria or overt nephropathy, both angiotensin-converting enzyme (ACE) inhibitors and angiotensin II receptor blockers (ARBs) have been shown to lower urinary protein excretion and slow the rate of disease progression.

- Randomized controlled trials of intensive therapies that resulted in average A1C values of 7% have found that every percentage point decrease in A1C is associated with significantly decreased rates of retinopathy, nephropathy, and neuropathy, with no threshold effect.

Macrovascular Disease

- All patients with diabetes who are older than 40 years should take aspirin (75-162 mg/d) for primary prevention of macrovascular disease, unless they have a specific contraindication to aspirin. In addition, all patients with diabetes who have a history of myocardial infarction, vascular bypass, stroke or transient ischemic attack, peripheral vascular disease, claudication, or angina should take a daily aspirin for secondary prevention.

- Statin therapy improves outcomes among patients with diabetes, including those without clinical evidence of coronary artery disease.

How do I talk to my patients about the complications of diabetes?

Discussing diabetes complications requires both sensitivity and honesty. It is important to offer hope by providing information about what can be done to prevent and treat these devastating problems, including concrete actions that patients can implement. One way to present the information is as a bad news/good news situation. The bad news is that complications can and do occur. The good news is that we know more about preventing and treating these complications than ever before.

- Most patients with type 2 diabetes are aware of the complications because of what they have been told by friends or family members with diabetes. Early in the course of their diabetes, ask patients what they know or have experienced in terms of the complications and what concerns or questions they have. Reassure patients that what happened to people with diabetes in the past is no longer inevitable.

- It is important to review the results of annual screenings with patients and explain what the findings mean in terms of their treatment and future health. *Your Diabetes Test Record* in Chapter 10 of the *Diabetes Care Guide Toolkit* can help patients focus on the importance of these findings. Patients should be encouraged to bring the form to their next visit and remind you when tests are due. An example of this tool, partially filled out, is shown in **Figure 12-1**.

- Use the professional education resources available on the Internet, such as the Diabetes Complications Risk Profile from the Michigan Diabetes Research and Training Center (http://med.umich.edu/mdrtc/ education/profedu.htm), to help patients understand the meaning of their screening results and adopt behaviors that may improve these results.

- While stressing the importance of glucose and blood pressure control to prevent complications, remember to point out that there are no guarantees. Let patients know, however, that they are increasing their odds and lowering their risks by doing all they can to care for their diabetes and their health. Provide patients with *The ABCs to Better Diabetes Care* from Chapter 10 of the *Diabetes Care Guide Toolkit*, which can help them achieve their goals.

- At the same time, avoid using the threat of complications as a method for encouraging behavior change. Scare tactics are ineffective for long-term behavior change.

Diabetic Retinopathy

Diabetic retinopathy is classified as nonproliferative (mild, moderate, or severe) and proliferative. Changes in retinal blood flow occur after several years of diabetes. These changes cause retinal ischemia, which in turn promotes growth factors that stimulate proliferation of new blood vessels that are more prone to leak blood. This process leads to scarring and fibrosis. As fibrous tissue contracts with time, it may put traction on the retina, causing retinal detachment with resultant vision loss. New vessels can also become more permeable and leak serum, which causes macular edema. Primary and secondary prevention of retinopathy involves optimal control of hyperglycemia, blood pressure, and lipids, as well as regularly scheduled dilated eye examinations.

Eye Examinations

All adults with diabetes should undergo an initial comprehensive, dilated eye examination by an ophthalmologist knowledgeable and experienced in diagnosing retinopathy and its management.

- Type 1 diabetes: Initial eye examination should occur within 1 year after the onset of diabetes.

- Type 2 diabetes: Initial eye examination should occur shortly after diagnosis.

All patients with diabetes should receive annual follow-up eye examinations by an ophthalmologist.

- More frequent evaluation is indicated if retinopathy is progressive.

- If the results of an examination are normal, the next examination may be scheduled less frequently (2 to 3 years) on the advice of an eye care professional.

Women with diabetes who are planning a pregnancy should receive a comprehensive eye

Name: *Mary Jones*

Year *2007–2008*

Tests	My Goal	3/15	4/30	6/15				My Notes
				Dates of Tests				
Weight	200	225	217	220				
Blood pressure	130/80	140/98	138/80	140/80				
A1C	*Less than 7.0*	9.5	8.6	8.2				
LDL	*Less than 100*	140	—	—				
HDL	*Greater than 50*	60						
Triglycerides	*Less than 150*	140	—	—				
Eye exam	*Yearly*							*Schedule my next exam for Dec. 2007*
Foot exam	*Yearly*							*Schedule my next exam for Jan. 2008*

Figure 12-1. **Diabetes Test Record** This figure shows a sample Diabetes Test Record (first tool in Chapter 10 of the toolkit) on which a patient has been recording her test results.

Ocular Telemedicine for Diabetic Retinopathy

Nearly half of adults with diabetes in the United States do not have eye examinations at the recommended frequency, which greatly limits early intervention. To reduce barriers to treatment, nonmydriatic digital retinal imaging telemedicine systems are being developed. These systems allow remote diagnosis of the clinical level of diabetic retinopathy and diabetic macular edema in a nonophthalmologic setting, which aids appropriate triage for eye care.

One such system is the Joslin Vision Network, a digital teleophthalmology system designed by the Joslin Diabetes Center in Boston, Massachusetts. Nonmydriatic digital color images of the retina and pertinent health information are forwarded to an image reading center for diagnosis and development of a treatment plan. In eyes that can be graded by this technique, the technique offers a very high correlation with dilated clinical examination by an ophthalmologist who specializes in retinal disease. When the Joslin Vision Network was implemented in a primary care setting to supplement an existing referral program for diabetes eye care, the annual diabetic retinopathy surveillance rate increased by nearly 50%.

examination and should be counseled on the risk of the development or progression of retinopathy. Transient retinopathy progression has been associated with intensification of glycemic control. For women with diabetes who are pregnant, a comprehensive eye examination is indicated during the first trimester. Close follow-up is indicated throughout pregnancy and up to 1 year postpartum. In addition, patients with pre-existing proteinuria need to be monitored closely because of the risk of worsening retinopathy.

A patient with any level of macular edema or severe nonproliferative or proliferative retinopathy should be referred to a retina specialist knowledgeable and experienced in the management of diabetic retinopathy. For a discussion of digital retinal imaging telemedicine systems, see *Ocular Telemedicine for Diabetic Retinopathy*.

Diabetic Nephropathy

Screening for Kidney Disease

Microalbuminuria—the presence of trace levels of albumin in the urine—is an indicator of early nephropathy. Albuminuria is also associated with a several-fold increase in cardiovascular disease in diabetes. Patients with diabetes should be screened annually for the presence of microalbuminuria.

- Type 1 diabetes: Annual screening should begin 5 years after the onset of diabetes.

- Type 2 diabetes: Annual screening should begin at diagnosis.

Screening can be initiated with a standard dipstick urinalysis; if no protein is detected, however, a more sensitive test for microalbuminuria should be performed.

- A random spot urine collection to determine the albumin-to-creatinine ratio is convenient and cost-effective and is the screening method preferred by the American Diabetes Association (ADA); a timed urine collection or 24-hour collection is rarely necessary. **Table 12-1** shows the classification of urine albumin excretion.

- Because of variability in albumin excretion, two of three specimens collected over 3 to 6 months should be abnormal before a patient is designated as having microalbuminuria. Febrile illness, exercise within the past 24 hours, infection, hematuria, menstruation, marked hyperglycemia, and marked hypertension can lead to elevations above baseline and false-positive results.

If a patient tests positive for microalbuminuria (or macroalbuminuria), a 24-hour urine sample for measurement of creatinine clearance and protein loss offers the most precise quantification of nephropathy. On a 24-hour urine sample, microalbuminuria is defined as a urinary albumin excretion of 30 mg/24 h or 20 µg/min. Overt nephropathy is diagnosed at a urine albumin excretion of greater than 300 mg/24 h; thereafter, the disease tends to progress, with a decline in the glomerular filtration rate (GFR) of

Table 12-1. Classification of Urine Albumin Excretion

Category	Spot Collection (µg/mg creatinine)
Normal	<30
Microalbuminuria	30–299
Macroalbuminuria (clinical albuminuria)	300

Reprinted with permission from: American Diabetes Association. Standards of medical care in diabetes—2006. Diabetes Care. 2006;29 Suppl 1:S4-42.

about 1 mL/min/1.73 m^2 each month. However, this course of progression can be reduced by optimal blood pressure control.

In addition to screening for microalbuminuria, the ADA recommends that all patients with diabetes—regardless of their degree of albumin excretion—have their serum creatinine levels measured for the estimation of GFR and the staging of chronic kidney disease (**Table 12-2**).

- Up to 30% of patients with type 2 diabetes may have a low GFR in the absence of significant microalbuminuria.

- A GFR below 60 mL/min/1.73 m^2 is a risk factor for the progression of renal disease and for cardiovascular events, even in the absence of albuminuria.

The Cockcroft-Gault and the Modification of Diet in Renal Disease (MDRD) study group equations calculate GFR based on serum creatinine, age, race, and gender. Either equation can be used. Laboratories often provide a calculated GFR with the creatinine level. A GFR calculator is available on the accompanying CD-ROM and on the ACP Diabetes Portal (`http://diabetes.acponline.org`).

Patients with a GFR below 60 mL/min/1.73 m^2 and patients with hypertension or hyperkalemia that is difficult to manage should be referred to a renal specialist.

Slowing the Progression of Kidney Disease

Several large-scale clinical trials have shown that nephropathy can be prevented or its progression delayed by interventions that provide

Table 12-2. Stages of Chronic Kidney Disease

Stage	Description	GFR (mL/min/ 1.73 m^2)
1	Kidney damage with normal or increased GFR	≥90
2	Kidney damage with mildly decreased GFR	60–89
3	Moderately decreased GFR	30–59
4	Severely decreased GFR	15–29
5	Kidney failure	<15 or dialysis

GFR = glomerular filtration rate.

Adapted with permission from: National Kidney Foundation Kidney Disease Outcome Quality Initiative (K/DOQI) Advisory Board. K/DOQI clinical practice guidelines for chronic kidney disease: evaluation, classification, and stratification. Available at: www.kidney.org/professionals/KDOQI/guidelines_ckd/toc.htm. Accessed 3 October 2006.

tight control of blood pressure and glucose levels. Much attention is therefore given to early detection and aggressive intervention in diabetic nephropathy. Tight glycemic control should be initiated at the onset of type 1 and type 2 diabetes.

Elevated blood pressure may have the greatest effect on the development of proteinuria and nephropathy. Whether specific antihypertensive agents improve proteinuria to a greater degree than the decrease in blood pressure alone remains controversial. Currently, the use of an ACE inhibitor or ARB is favored. However, studies of beta-blockers, thiazides, and other classes of antihypertension drugs have also shown favorable responses. Whether all patients with diabetes, regardless of whether they have hypertension, should begin therapy with an ACE inhibitor or an ARB before the onset of microalbuminuria requires further study.

Decreasing dietary protein to less than 0.8 g/kg of body weight daily has been shown to have a salutary effect on creatinine clearance and proteinuria. However, dietary protein restriction is one of the most difficult strategies for treating nephropathy. Such regimens are complex, are difficult for most patients to implement, and may decrease overall adherence to the meal plan. In addition, the higher amounts of carbohydrates and fat that a protein-restricted diet requires may be a concern.

Peripheral Vascular Disease and Diabetic Foot Ulcers

Peripheral vascular disease (PVD) disproportionately affects the elderly as well as non-Hispanic blacks and Mexican-Americans. Diabetic vascular disease is often complicated by the presence of peripheral neuropathy, which increases the risk for developing traumatic foot ulcers. The cost of managing foot ulcers in patients with diabetes is estimated to approach $28,000 for the 2 years after the onset of the diagnosis of the foot ulcer. In addition, survival is significantly reduced in patients with diabetic foot ulcers.

Foot Examinations

A comprehensive foot examination should be performed annually in all patients with diabetes to identify high-risk foot problems. Signs in patient examination rooms reminding those with diabetes to remove their shoes can greatly facilitate this examination. The foot examination should include:

- Visual inspection for deformities of the toes, arch, and nails

- Skin examination to detect calluses, fungal infection, ulcers, or wounds

- Neuropathy assessment using a tuning fork to test vibratory sensation and a Semmes-Weinstein 5.07 (10-g) monofilament to test light touch

- Assessment of pedal pulses

Foot Sensory Exam Findings is an illustrated worksheet in Chapter 12 of the *Diabetes Care Guide Toolkit* that enables you to mark up the results of filament tests for 10 visits. An illustrated tutorial on how to use a monofilament is available on the ACP Diabetes Portal at http://diabetes.acponline.org.

Early recognition of PVD and peripheral neuropathy are the best tools to prevent amputations. Signs of diabetic vascular disease include claudication, loss of foot hair, delayed capillary filling, dependent rubor, and absence of peripheral pulses. The ankle to brachial index (ABI) correlates well with the presence of arterial occlusive disease. The ABI should be measured in patients with symptoms of PVD and in asymptomatic patients with diminished pedal pulses on palpation and other physical signs of vascular insufficiency. The ABI is calculated by measuring systolic blood pressure in the posterior tibial and dorsalis pedis arteries of both lower extremities. The highest of these four measurements is used for the ankle pressure. Pressure is also measured in both brachial arteries, with the highest of the two used as the brachial pressure. The ratio is then calculated as:

ABI = ankle pressure/brachial pressure

The interpretation of ABI results is shown in **Table 12-3**. In patients with values above 0.9 but in whom PVD is still suspected, an ABI can be calculated after a treadmill test. If the ABI decreases 20% or more following exercise, PVD is very likely present. Patients with abnormal ABIs should be further assessed and treated for cardiovascular risk factors. Those with moderate or advanced ischemia should be referred to a vascular specialist for further evaluation.

The classification of diabetic foot ulcers is shown in **Table 12-4**. For patients with foot ulcers or high-risk foot conditions or with a history of ulcers or amputation, a multidisciplinary team approach is beneficial, including infectious disease, podiatry and/or orthopedic surgery, vascular surgery, endocrinology, and rehabilitation specialists.

Foot Care Education

All patients with diabetes need education regarding routine self-care practices and the avoidance of smoking. Emphasize that caring for their feet is one of the least expensive and easiest things they can do in caring for their diabetes and that it can have a very real benefit in preventing amputations.

Basic foot care education includes the importance of looking at the feet daily (after a shower or when getting undressed) for signs of injury, blisters, or damage from poorly fitting shoes and

Table 12-3. Interpretation of Ankle-Brachial Index

Ankle-Brachial Index	Interpretation
>1.3	Noncompressible calcified arteries
1.0–1.3	Normal
0.4–0.9	Moderate arterial obstruction, often with claudication
<0.4	Advanced ischemia

Table 12-4. Classification of Diabetic Foot Ulcers

Grade	Description
Grade 0	No ulcer in a high-risk foot
Grade 1	Superficial ulcer involving a full skin thickness but not underlying tissues
Grade 2	Deep ulcer penetrating down to ligaments and muscle but no bone involvement or abscess formation
Grade 3	Deep ulcer with cellulitis or abscess formation, often with osteomyelitis
Grade 4	Localized gangrene
Grade 5	Extensive gangrene involving the whole foot

the need to protect the feet by wearing appropriate footwear. Offer a podiatry referral for patients who have difficulty caring for their toenails or who have corns or calluses that need treatment.

Patients with signs of nerve damage need more specific information. During the examination, point out areas of decreased sensation that the patient needs to inspect closely on a daily basis. Patients may benefit from a referral for podiatry services for routine foot care services or orthotics. One pair of shoes per year is generally a covered benefit for patients with neuropathy.

🖐 *Taking Care of Your Feet* in Chapter 12 of the *Diabetes Care Guide Toolkit* provides instructions for proper foot care that all patients with diabetes should follow.

Coronary Artery Disease in Diabetes

Persons with diabetes have a greatly increased risk of cardiovascular disease. The increased risk seen in the MRFIT trial was present even after adjusting for age and other cardiovascular risk factors, such as smoking, hypertension, and hypercholesterolemia. In those with multiple risk factors, the increase in cardiovascular risk was even greater. In a study carried out in Finland, the risk of death from coronary artery disease for persons with diabetes who had not had a prior myocardial infarction was comparable to that of persons without diabetes who had already had a prior myocardial infarction. These results provided the rationale for considering the presence of diabetes to be a coronary artery disease equivalent in the National Cholesterol Education Program. Persons with diabetes are thus classified in the highest cardiovascular risk category, regardless of the presence of established coronary artery disease.

Screening Cardiac Stress Tests

Guidelines on screening cardiac stress tests vary, and no consensus currently exists. The ADA currently recommends screening cardiac stress testing in patients with diabetes who also have any of the characteristics below:

- A history of peripheral or carotid occlusive disease

- A sedentary lifestyle, age 35 years or older, and the intention of beginning a vigorous exercise program

- Two or more of the following cardiovascular risk factors: dyslipidemia, hypertension, smoking, a positive family history of premature coronary disease, and the presence of microalbuminuria or macroalbuminuria

Remember that sudden exercise in sedentary subjects can precipitate myocardial infarction. Most experts agree that a complete physical examination and an exercise stress test should be performed in patients with type 1 diabetes who are older than 35 years and have had diabetes for more than 10 years.

Abnormal results on a stress test in an asymptomatic patient need to be evaluated on an individual basis. All patients should be treated for risk factors of coronary artery disease according to currently established guidelines for high-risk patients, including lipid and blood pressure

intervention. In addition, all patients should begin aspirin therapy if they are not already on it. Patients should be reinterviewed for atypical symptoms and referred to a cardiologist for consideration of invasive studies if noninvasive studies reveal major abnormalities.

Diabetic Peripheral Neuropathy

Up to 50% of patients with peripheral neuropathy experience symptoms, with pain being the most common. Peripheral sensory neuropathies vary in their presentation, but they typically begin with dysesthesias distally and symmetrically. They then progress to varying degrees of discomfort and numbness as they ascend symmetrically from the lower extremities. The sensory neuropathies can involve the upper extremities as well, but typically only after involvement in the lower extremities is severe, often up to the knee or above.

Sensory neuropathies are detected by testing vibration sense, pinprick, light touch, proprioception, and position sense. Use of the 10-g monofilament test is additionally recommended because an abnormal response to this test also identifies a foot at risk of ulceration. Patients must be informed about the degree of their neuropathic impairment, especially if it includes significant loss of vibratory or pain sensation, because they may not respond rapidly to burn or skin-breaking injury. Pointing out specific areas during the examination is a particularly useful educational strategy.

Painful peripheral sensory neuropathy is an exceptionally difficult problem for which there are no consistently effective therapies. Approximately 10% of patients with diabetic peripheral neuropathy experience persistent pain. Diabetic neuropathic pain can interfere with quality of life by affecting mood, coordination, walking, the ability to work, and the ability to manage other aspects of diabetes and health. It is often worse at night. If pain persists for more than 3 months, it is unlikely to resolve spontaneously. Pain that lasts more than 6 months is classified as chronic.

Management of Painful Neuropathy

Treatment of diabetic neuropathic pain is largely symptomatic. Modification of risk factors (glycemia, hypertension, hyperlipidemia, obesity, and smoking) may help prevent neuropathy.

The ADA recommends a stepwise approach to the symptomatic treatment of painful neuropathy:

- Stabilization of glycemic control

- First-line treatment: tricyclic antidepressants

- Second-line treatment: antiepileptic drugs

- Third-line treatment: opioid or opioid-like drugs

- Fourth-line treatment: possible referral to a pain clinic

Antidepressants

Duloxetine is the only antidepressant officially approved by the U.S. Food and Drug Administration (FDA) for use in diabetic peripheral neuropathy. It is a selective serotonin and norepinephrine reuptake inhibitor. Common side effects include nausea, somnolence, dizziness, constipation, dry mouth, increased sweating, decreased appetite, and asthenia.

Tricyclic antidepressants are not officially approved by the FDA for diabetic peripheral neuropathy, but they may help some patients. However, the side effect profile of these drugs (including orthostatic hypotension, drowsiness, constipation, urinary retention, and dry mouth) needs to be considered when prescribing these medications.

Antiepileptic Agents

Pregabalin is the only antiepileptic drug approved for use in diabetic peripheral neuropathy. Adverse effects include dizziness, somnolence, peripheral edema, nausea, and weight gain. No known drug interactions are associated with the use of pregabalin.

Other antiepileptic drugs used to treat painful neuropathy include carbamazepine, gabapentin, lamotrigine, sodium valproate, and topiramate. Studies evaluating the efficacy of these drugs have been small and not always conclusive; hence, these drugs have not been officially approved by the FDA for this use.

Opioid or Opioid-like Drugs

Third-line treatment for diabetic painful neuropathy includes the use of opioid or opioid-like drugs, such as oxycodone and tramadol. Referral to a pain clinic is recommended before prescribing these medications. Combinations of medications—for example, morphine and gabapentin—sometimes help to reduce the pain.

Other Agents

Alpha-lipoic acid (600 mg/d for periods ranging from weeks to months) has been associated with an improvement in symptoms and in neurologic deficits, but this drug has not been approved by the FDA. It is sold in health food stores and on the Internet as a dietary supplement. This agent appears to be safe.

Mononeuropathies and Multifocal Neuropathies

Some mononeuropathies are not specific to diabetes and are not thought to be related to the duration of diabetes. Their primary symptom is usually acute local discomfort, with abnormal conduction that corresponds to the distribution of a single nerve, multiple peripheral nerves, the brachial or lumbosacral plexus, or nerve roots. Focal neuropathies, such as lateral femoral cutaneous nerve palsy, are more common in middle-aged patients or those with sensorimotor polyneuropathy. No specific strategies detect or prevent focal neuropathies.

Diabetic mononeuropathies can involve the median (carpal tunnel syndrome) and ulnar (wrist drop) nerves, the sciatic or femoral nerves (foot drop), or the third, fourth, or sixth cranial nerves (paralysis). They have no clear precipitant or treatment, and they usually resolve spontaneously in weeks. Radiculopathy of the chest or abdomen can mimic herpes zoster. In rare cases, when more than one nerve is involved simultaneously, the condition is termed "mononeuropathy multiplex," indicating that each affected nerve is independently involved. Patients with long-standing diabetes and vasculopathy may develop diabetic amyotrophy, which involves pain, atrophy, and fasciculations of the limb girdle muscles.

Autonomic Neuropathies

Cardiovascular Autonomic Neuropathy

The development of diabetic autonomic neuropathy is clinically challenging to treat and an important indicator of patients who are at very high risk for cardiovascular disease and sudden death. Cardiovascular neuropathies may result in orthostatic hypotension, a lack of normal variation of the heart rate with breathing, tachycardia, and sudden death. To treat orthostatic hypotension, fludrocortisone and midodrine are the drugs of first choice. Patients being treated with these drugs should be closely monitored for supine hypertension, abnormal potassium levels, and fluid retention.

Gastrointestinal Autonomic Neuropathy

Gastrointestinal autonomic neuropathy includes gastroparesis and diarrhea. Gastroparesis may present with bloating, early satiety, vomiting, or symptoms of gastroesophageal reflux disease. Diabetic diarrhea is characteristically nocturnal but can occur at any time of the day and may alternate with constipation. Treatment is largely targeted at symptoms and includes the use of metoclopramide for gastroparesis.

Screening for Autonomic Neuropathies

All patients with type 2 diabetes and those who have had type 1 diabetes for more than 5 years should be screened for autonomic neuropathy by history and physical examination directed at the cardiovascular and gastrointestinal systems. Postural changes in blood pressure should be monitored yearly. Any patients with unexplained postural symptoms, such as dizziness on standing and syncope, can be referred for additional laboratory studies and testing for autonomic neuropathy.

Erectile Dysfunction

Erectile dysfunction is one of the more common autonomic neuropathies of diabetes and has historically tended to be underdiagnosed. More than 50% of men with diabetes are believed to have some degree of erectile dysfunction after 10 years with the disease. Furthermore, erectile dysfunction may be a marker for other, more serious vascular disease or neurologic dysfunction. In the erectile dysfunction of diabetes, nocturnal and morning erections are characteristically absent.

Oral therapies for erectile dysfunction, which help sustain a normal erection in many men with diabetes, include the phosphodiesterase type 5 (PDE-5) inhibitors sildenafil, vardenafil, and tadalafil. These drugs are nearly as effective in the presence of diabetes as in its absence. Before they are prescribed for patients with diabetes, however, other causes of erectile dysfunction, including hypogonadism, depression, and advanced vascular disease, should be ruled out. No side effects are specific to diabetes. However, these agents should be avoided in patients with significant cardiovascular disease. They can potentiate the hypotensive effects of nitrate, and they are contraindicated in patients who are using organic nitrates in any form—whether regularly or intermittently—or alpha-adrenergic receptor blockers. In patients with more advanced erectile dysfunction or those failing to respond to PDE-5 inhibitors, intracavernosal injections of vasodilators or penile implants offer the best hope.

Screening for Erectile Dysfunction

Screening for erectile dysfunction should include taking a thorough history to detect loss of libido or other signs and symptoms of hormonal deficiency; underlying psychological issues affect-ing sexual relationships, including depression; and possible use of drugs that adversely affect sexual function.

Sexual Dysfunction in Women

Several small studies have evaluated sexual function in women with type 1 diabetes. Most have found a higher risk of sexual dysfunction (e.g., decreased sexual arousal) and the need for further study in these patients.

13. Diabetes in Women of Childbearing Age

Planning for Pregnancy

Babies born to mothers with either type 1 or type 2 diabetes have a higher risk of major congenital malformations, which lead to increased morbidity and mortality. Tight control of blood glucose during the pre-conception period and the first trimester of pregnancy can significantly reduce the rate of malformations. Given that two thirds of the pregnancies in women with diabetes are unplanned, you will need to counsel patients on pre-conception planning if they are of childbearing age.

- Counseling should begin at age 12 or 13 years.

- Counseling should emphasize the importance of planning for pregnancy for the best possible outcomes.

The multidisciplinary team needed to manage diabetes in women who desire pregnancy should include a diabetologist, the primary care physician, an obstetrician familiar with diabetes management of high-risk pregnancies, a diabetes educator, a nutritionist, and a social worker.

Glycemic Goals

Epidemiologic studies have shown that in women with diabetes, lowering the hemoglobin A1C value to within 1% of normal decreases the risk of congenital malformation and spontaneous abortion to a level close to that of women without diabetes. Thus, the goal should be to achieve blood glucose levels as near to normal as possible before conception and throughout the pregnancy, without undue risk of hypoglycemia. Optimum glycemic goals that your patient should aim for during pregnancy are shown in **Table 13-1**.

Management of Diabetes Before and During Pregnancy

Evaluation

The management of diabetes in women of childbearing age who want to become pregnant should ideally start before conception and continue throughout the pregnancy.

- Medical and obstetrical history should include an evaluation to detect the presence of complications associated with diabetes and of other coexisting medical conditions.

- Physical examination should include a dilated eye examination by an ophthalmologist, a cardiovascular assessment (electrocardiogram, echocardiogram, or cardiac stress test, depending on risk), and a neurologic examination. A complete gynecologic examination, including a Pap smear, is recommended before conception.

- Laboratory evaluation should include assessment of glycemic control, thyroid function, and indices of complications of diabetes that may deteriorate during pregnancy, such as serum creatinine level and spot urine albumin-to-creatinine ratio (to detect microalbuminuria).

Medical Management

Strategies to achieve glycemic and other goals in pregnant women are somewhat different from those in other patients with diabetes.

- Insulin should replace oral hypoglycemic agents or other injectable agents whose safety is not established during pregnancy.

- The safety of glargine, a long-acting analogue of insulin, is similarly not established during pregnancy. Therefore, patients who are

Table 13-1. Glycemic Goals During Pregnancy

Type of Diabetes	Blood Glucose
Preexisting diabetes Fasting and pre-meal 1-hour post-meal or peak postprandial	60–99 mg/dL 100–129 mg/dL
Gestational diabetes Fasting 1-hour post-meal	<100 mg/dL <130 mg/dL

Adapted from Joslin Diabetes Center and Diabetes Clinic. Guideline for detection and management of diabetes in pregnancy. 9/15/05. Available at www.joslin.org/Files/ Gest_guide.pdf. Accessed 3 October 2006.

planning a pregnancy or who are pregnant should be taken off glargine.

- Angiotensin-converting enzyme (ACE) inhibitors, angiotensin II receptor blockers (ARBs), and cholesterol-lowering drugs should be stopped before pregnancy. Other medications should be checked and, if not known to be safe during pregnancy, replaced.

- Women with diabetes who are contemplating pregnancy or are pregnant should be referred to a diabetes educator and nutritionist for counseling regarding self-monitoring of blood glucose and medical nutrition therapy.

- Regular exercise should be encouraged, especially after meals, to improve postprandial hyperglycemia.

What do women of childbearing age with diabetes need to know about conception and pregnancy?

The following information should be shared with women of childbearing age with diabetes:

- Achieving blood glucose control as close to normal as possible before attempting to conceive and avoiding erratic daily blood glucose levels are essential. This message needs to be conveyed to all female patients when they reach childbearing age (usually age 13 years).

- Effective contraception should be used until good blood glucose control is achieved (A1C value of 6%–7%).

- Women with diabetes nowadays are more likely to have a healthy baby than in the past.

Although risks for congenital anomalies and other fetal and neonatal complications of maternal diabetes are present, these risks are reduced to the level of women without diabetes if blood glucose levels are normalized before a patient becomes pregnant.

- Review the effects of pregnancy on maternal complications of diabetes.

- Discuss the risks of obstetrical complications in women with diabetes.

- Educate patients on the increased care demands of diabetes during pregnancy.

- Make patients aware of the risk for diabetes in the child.

- Women with gestational diabetes need to be screened for diabetes early in any subsequent pregnancies.

Complications of Diabetes During Pregnancy

Retinopathy

During pregnancy, the risk of accelerated diabetic retinopathy is increased. A baseline comprehensive eye examination and appropriate treatment are thus necessary before conception. Women need to be educated about the risk of the development and progression of diabetic retinopathy during pregnancy.

Nephropathy

Serum creatinine and spot urine values should be measured before conception. Women with a severe decline in renal function (serum creatinine >3 mg/dL or creatinine clearance <50 mL/min/1.73 m²) are at high risk of a permanent decline in renal function. In women with less severe renal insufficiency, the decline in renal function is transient. Proteinuria of 190 mg/24 h or more, before or during pregnancy, is associated with a 3-fold increased risk of a hypertensive disorder in the second half of pregnancy. Women with diabetes should be counseled on the risk of impaired renal function developing and progressing during pregnancy.

Neuropathy

Both autonomic and peripheral neuropathies should be identified before conception and followed closely for exacerbation. The presence of an autonomic neuropathy in the form of gastroparesis, orthostatic hypotension, hypoglycemic unawareness, or urinary retention can complicate diabetes management. Compartment syndromes (e.g., carpal tunnel syndrome) may be exacerbated during pregnancy.

Cardiovascular Disease

The American Diabetes Association recommends assessment and treatment of cardiovascular disease before conception in patients with diabetes. Untreated cardiovascular disease increases the risk of mortality during pregnancy in these patients.

Hypertension

Women with diabetes have an increased risk of pregnancy-induced hypertension. This risk is higher when proteinuria in excess of 190 mg/dL is present before conception or during pregnancy. Aggressive control of blood pressure should be employed to avoid worsening of nephropathy and retinopathy. ACE inhibitors, ARBs, and diuretics should be avoided in women with diabetes who are planning to become pregnant and should be stopped as soon as possible in cases of unplanned pregnancy. Antihypertensive agents that can be safely used during pregnancy include alpha-methyldopa, beta-blockers (except atenolol), calcium channel blockers, and hydralazine.

14. Diabetes in Elderly Patients

As the population lives longer, the number of older adults with diabetes will continue to increase significantly. In addition to macro- and microvascular complications of diabetes, elderly patients with diabetes are also at increased risk of the adverse effects of polypharmacy, functional disabilities, cognitive dysfunction, depression, urinary incontinence, falls, and persistent pain.

Elderly patients with diabetes represent a heterogeneous population ranging from those who are highly functional and reside independently in the community, to those who live in assisted-care facilities, to functionally dependent persons who live in nursing homes. Although the overall goals of diabetes management in the elderly are similar to those in younger adults, several concerns are unique and need individualized consideration.

The ideal care of elderly patients with diabetes requires a multidisciplinary team approach that includes a diabetologist, a primary care physician and/or gerontologist, a nurse educator, a nutritionist, an exercise physiologist, and a social worker. Diabetes education is a covered benefit by Medicare, and elderly patients should be referred for diabetes education and medical nutrition therapy. Individual education can be provided for patients who have hearing or other impairments if the referral specifies that need. Many community and senior citizens centers have programs that help persons with diabetes, such as exercise and healthy eating programs. Maintaining a current list of these resources will allow you to provide this information to patients when it is needed.

Because older adults may have hearing, cognitive, or other impairments, assess their understanding at the end of each visit or educational session by using the "teach-back" method—ask the patient to tell you in his or her own words what advice he or she received and what actions will be taken at home to implement it.

Glycemic Goals and Control of Other Risk Factors

Glycemic goals in elderly patients with diabetes should be established in light of overall health, coexisting conditions, and life expectancy. A highly functional elderly patient may be able to use a complicated regimen and achieve tight hemoglobin A1C control. On the other hand, a higher A1C goal may be appropriate for a functionally impaired or frail elderly patient, or one with multiple chronic illnesses that also require self-management. Glycemic goals should be periodically reassessed in this population because declining health in an elderly patient may require upward adjustment of a goal set when the patient was in better health.

Because of the higher risk of post-meal hyperglycemia in elderly patients, normal fasting glucose levels may be accompanied by high A1C results. A practical approach to treatment is for these patients to use walking or other low-impact exercise and modest dietary modifications, taking care to avoid inappropriate weight loss, combined with self-monitoring of blood glucose that includes postprandial readings.

The goals for management of risk factors in elderly patients are similar to those in young adults. However, additional factors, such as renal dysfunction, coexisting medical conditions, polypharmacy, and drug-to-drug interactions, should be considered and may lead to less strict control. There is strong evidence suggesting a reduction of morbidity and mortality by tight control of blood pressure in elderly patients with diabetes. The evidence is less convincing for tight control of lipid lowering, glycemic control, and aspirin use in this population.

Medical Management

Oral diabetes medications, alone or in combination, are prescribed for elderly patients without specific restrictions. However, the following cautions should be noted:

- Coexisting medical conditions and liver function should be carefully evaluated before selecting medications.

- Renal function should be followed because elderly patients may have normal serum creatinine levels, even if creatinine clearance is low, as a result of their lower muscle mass.

- The sulfonylurea class of drugs should be used with caution because of its tendency to cause hypoglycemia.

- Unintended weight loss and gastrointestinal side effects are limiting factors for the use of metformin.

- Newer agents, such as exenatide (Byetta) and pramlintide (Symlin), are not well studied in this population.

Diet and Exercise

Dietary modifications may have a limited role in the management of diabetes in elderly patients. Many factors may be involved, including the difficulty in changing a lifetime of eating habits, limitations in the patient's ability to cook or shop for groceries, dependence on family or others for cooking and shopping, decreased appetite, other health issues, and financial concerns. In addition, weight loss can increase morbidity and mortality in the elderly. Weight should be assessed at each visit, with a focus on unintentional weight loss.

Modest dietary modifications that avoid large fluctuations in blood sugars without undue risk of weight loss and nutritional deficiency can be a reasonable goal. Encouraging patients to eat small meals at frequent intervals or to use simple meal planning methods, such as the plate method or healthy food choices (see Chapter 5, Helping Patients Make Lifestyle Changes), is often adequate. Older adults who aim for tight glucose control will benefit from a referral to a dietitian to develop a personal meal plan.

Exercise is beneficial for the elderly, not only for improved glycemic control, but also for muscle strengthening, gait and balance, and overall quality of life. No additional screening for cardiovascular disease is needed when starting low-impact exercise as tolerated; however, cardiac clearance should be sought before starting an intensive exercise program. Examples of activities appropriate for older adults include low-impact exercises (walking, swimming) and weight training. Many community and senior centers have exercise programs specifically for older adults. The Centers for Disease Control and Prevention's program "Growing Stronger" (available at: `www.cdc.gov/nccdphp/dnpa/physical/growing_stronger/index.htm`) is a guide to strength training for older adults.

Special Considerations

Hypoglycemia

Hypoglycemia is a serious complication of diabetes management in elderly patients. This complication increases the risk of cardiovascular events (myocardial ischemia, angina), stroke, impaired cognition, and falls in the elderly. Older adults are also more likely to experience neurologic symptoms of hypoglycemia, such as dizziness, weakness, delirium, and confusion, as opposed to the adrenergic symptoms of tremor, palpitations, and sweating that are commonly seen in younger adults. Consequently, hypoglycemic episodes in an elderly patient may remain undiagnosed or be misdiagnosed as a primary neurologic event.

Hypoglycemia can be a particularly frightening event for older adults, and they may choose to omit oral medications or insulin rather than risk a reaction. Outcomes of even a mild episode of hypoglycemia can be poor in an elderly patient. For example, hypoglycemia causing dizziness or weakness in a frail elderly person may cause a fall and subsequent injury, requiring nursing home placement. The risk of hypoglycemia can also limit a patient's independence and ability to live alone or take advantage of social opportunities.

Patients and their families or caregivers need instruction on the recognition, treatment, and prevention of hypoglycemia. These issues are addressed more fully in Chapter 6 (Monitoring Glycemic Control). Because the symptoms among older adults may be different from those listed in the typical educational handout, this information needs to be personalized and reviewed carefully with the patient, family, and caregivers. In addition, recommend that patients keep glucose tablets or a juice box by their bed to help prevent falls if hypoglycemia occurs at night. Wearing medical identification is particularly important for this age group.

Nonketotic Hyperosmolar Syndrome

Elderly patients with diabetes have a greater risk of developing a nonketotic hyperosmolar state because of their higher risk of dehydration. Adequate hydration is important to prevent this complication in elderly patients, especially during illnesses. Patients and their families need information about sick day management and the symptoms of nonketotic hyperosmolar syndrome.

Cognitive Impairment and Depression

Elderly persons with diabetes have a higher risk of cognitive dysfunction than do their peers without diabetes. In the early stages, most impairment is undiagnosed. Elderly patients with dementia are at higher risk for poor self-management, poor diabetes control, and complications of treatment (e.g., hypoglycemia). Early recognition of dementia will help you set

appropriate treatment goals (e.g., a higher A1C value) and avoid complicated treatment regimens. Elderly persons with diabetes also have a high risk of depression, and untreated depression is associated with poor glycemic control. Treatment of depression not only improves the patient's ability to manage his or her diabetes, but also improves quality of life. Cognitive impairment and depression in diabetes are addressed in more detail in Chapter 11 (Depression and Cognitive Dysfunction).

Polypharmacy

Whereas many—if not most—patients with type 2 diabetes take multiple medications for control of hypertension, hyperlipidemia, and hyperglycemia, the number of comorbid conditions requiring medications and the risks of drug interactions expands greatly in the elderly. Review these patients' medications regularly to assess for side effects, drug interactions, and the continued necessity of each medication. The cost of even the co-payments for the number of medications needed by these patients can be a limiting factor in their ability to take their prescribed medications.

Careful assessment of the medications being taken is needed at each visit to determine whether financial or other issues are affecting safe medication use (e.g., side effects; confusion about dosage/timing; use of over-the-counter, herbal, and vitamin preparations). Tips to help your patients manage their oral medications are included in Chapters 7 (Oral Diabetes Drugs) and 10 (Hyperlipidemia and Hypertension). In Chapter 7 of the *Diabetes Care Guide Toolkit* is a form where your patients can keep vital information regarding their medications handy at all times.

Falls

Falls are common in elderly patients with diabetes. The etiology of a fall is usually multifactorial and includes peripheral or autonomic neuropathy, drug adverse effects, nutritional deficiency, functional disability and muscle deconditioning, loss of vision, and coexisting conditions such as osteoarthritis.

Reversible causes of falls should be identified and treated. Intervention strategies that may reduce the risk of falls include supervised exercise programs, physical/occupational therapy, vision and hearing aids, and avoidance of medications that cause delirium, drowsiness, or confusion. Simple strategies that patients or their caregivers can use include adequate lighting, well-fitting footwear, avoidance of clutter, and placement of night lights in hallways and bathrooms.

Management of Elderly Patients in the Chronic Care Setting

Elderly persons living in an assisted-care or a nursing home setting have unique needs and problems. Overall health, life expectancy, and patient preference should guide management of these patients. Use of a regular diet may improve quality of life and prevent weight loss and so is the recommended meal plan in these settings. Exercise as tolerated remains important for these patients.

15. Diabetes in Specific Ethnic Groups

Risk and Complications of Diabetes

Several ethnic groups, including Hispanic Americans, African Americans, Asian Americans, Native Americans, and Pacific Islanders, have a higher prevalence of type 2 diabetes, impaired glucose intolerance, and gestational diabetes than white Americans have. Diabetes-related morbidity and mortality is also higher in these groups. Several theories have been proposed to explain these differences:

- The theory of the "thrifty genotype" suggests that some ethnic groups had a selective survival advantage in times of famine by having a highly efficient caloric storage system. In times of abundance, however, this feature becomes detrimental and predisposes to diabetes.

- Studies comparing migrant populations (e.g., Asian Americans) with native nonmigrant populations have shown an increased risk of diabetes in the migrant populations, which suggests an influence of environmental changes and western lifestyle. A diet high in fat and low in fiber, lack of exercise, and obesity are therefore being studied as causative factors for the higher prevalence of diabetes in various ethnic groups.

- Socioeconomic factors may also influence the prevalence of diabetes.

Ethnicity also affects the prevalence of diabetes-related complications:

- End-stage renal disease and diabetic retinopathy occur frequently in all of the ethnic groups previously listed (Hispanic Americans, African Americans, Asian Americans, Native Americans, Pacific Islanders).

- Hispanic Americans, African Americans, and Native Americans have higher rates of proteinuria than do white Americans.

- African Americans have higher rates of peripheral vascular disease and amputations than do other ethnic groups.

- Diabetes-related mortality rates are higher in Hispanic Americans, African Americans, and Native Americans than in other ethnic groups.

- Complication rates for Asian Americans vary according to country of ancestry.

Approach to Management

Diabetes should be considered a public health problem in these ethnic groups. Specific interventional strategies are being studied; in the meantime, the following general approaches to providing diabetes care should be followed:

- Persons belonging to any of the ethnic groups listed (Hispanic Americans, African Americans, Asian Americans, Native Americans, Pacific Islanders) should be screened for diabetes as high-risk persons.

- Patients of all ethnic groups need to be assessed for the impact of cultural and religious practices on diabetes care. Ask, "Do any of your religious or cultural beliefs or practices influence the way you care for your diabetes?"

- Diabetes education should be provided and programs developed that are culturally sensitive to language, literature, cultural beliefs, and values for both specific and diverse groups of patients.

- Educational materials should reflect the culture of the patient in terms of pictures, language, word usage, and food.

- Cultural attitudes toward food, obesity, and exercise need to be assessed and taken into account.

- Because different cultural groups may interpret information differently, assess understanding at the end of each visit or educational session by using the "teach-back" method—ask the patient to tell you in his or her own words what advice he or she received and what actions will be taken at home to implement it.

- A useful resource for tips on providing medical care to persons of various ethnic groups (not diabetes-specific) can be found at the following Web site: `http://med.umich.edu/multicultural/ccp/culture.htm`.

16. Emergencies in Diabetes

All persons involved in the care of persons with diabetes need to be able to determine when hospitalization is warranted. General hospital admission guidelines for diabetes are summarized in **Table 16-1**. When counseling patients about hypoglycemia and hyperglycemia, emphasize that the best treatment is prevention: be proactive by recognizing the signs early, be prepared to treat, treat appropriately, and seek prompt attention when needed. It is always better to err on the side of safety.

Hyperglycemia

Outpatient Management

Milder forms of hyperglycemia can often be treated in the outpatient setting. Testing for ketones (blood or urinary) is recommended in the following settings:

- When the blood glucose level is more than 250 mg/dL for two tests in a row

- During illness or infection

- After trauma or stressors

- When symptoms compatible with ketoacidosis, such as nausea, vomiting, or abdominal pain, are present

Persons with more pronounced insulin deficiency (see Table 17-2) are at highest risk of developing ketoacidosis. If a patient with small ketonuria (2+) experiences no altered level of consciousness, can monitor his or her blood sugars (every 1–2 hours for rapid analogues or 2–3 hours for regular insulin), administer insulin appropriately, and ingest fluids without difficulty, he or she can often be treated at home by following predetermined sick day rules. Even a patient with moderate ketonuria (3+) can often be treated at home with direct guidance from the diabetes care team.

The ability to absorb subcutaneous insulin is related to the level of hydration. If dehydration progresses at a rate that cannot be easily managed by oral intake, intravenous fluids will be required, regardless of the results of ketone testing, and intravenous insulin should also be considered. In the setting of large ketonuria (4+), more intensive monitoring is required, and hospitalization is encouraged, even if the patient reports feeling well.

Inpatient Management

The subtleties of hospital management of hyperglycemic emergencies are beyond the scope of this text and are reviewed elsewhere (see *Suggested Readings*). In general, the initial treatment plan for hyperglycemic emergencies includes stabilizing hemodynamic values, replenishing volume, administering insulin, correcting electrolyte abnormalities, and searching for precipitating causes. Intravenous insulin infusion is usually the preferred method of insulin delivery in an emergency because dehydration may be severe (decreasing subcutaneous absorption). Rapid titration of insulin may be required.

After the metabolic abnormalities have been corrected and the patient is ready to be transferred to subcutaneous administration of insulin (usually when the patient starts eating), intravenous and subcutaneous insulin administration need to be overlapped to avoid rebound ketoacidosis. Give short-acting or rapid-acting insulins 1 to 2 hours or intermediate or long-acting insulins 2 to 3 hours before terminating the insulin infusion to ensure adequate overlap.

What do I need to tell patients about hyperglycemia?

- Review when to test for ketones.

- Ensure that patients have in their home sufficient ketone-testing supplies, which can usually be purchased without a prescription. (The

Table 16-1. Hospital Admission Guidelines for Diabetes

Life-threatening acute metabolic complications of diabetes
   Diabetic ketoacidosis: Plasma glucose >250 mg/dL with arterial pH <7.30, serum bicarbonate <15 meq/L, and moderate ketonuria and/or ketonemia
   Hyperglycemic hyperosmolar state: Impaired mental status, usually with plasma glucose >600 mg/dL and elevated serum osmolality (>320 mosm/kg)
   Hypoglycemia with neuroglycopenia:
   • Blood glucose <50 mg/dL without rapid recovery of sensorium with treatment; *or*
   • Coma, seizures, or altered behavior due to documented or suspected hypoglycemia; *or*
   • Hypoglycemia has been treated but a responsible adult cannot observe the patient for the ensuing 12 hours; *or*
   • Expected prolonged hypoglycemia from medication such as sulfonylurea or long-acting insulin.
Newly diagnosed diabetes in children and adolescents*
Substantial and chronic poor metabolic control that necessitates close monitoring of the patient to determine the etiology of the control problem, with subsequent modification of therapy:
   • Hyperglycemia with volume depletion
   • Persistent refractory hyperglycemia associated with metabolic deterioration
   • Recurrent fasting hyperglycemia (>300 mg/dL) or A1C >2 times normal
   • Frequent swings between hypoglycemia <50 mg/dL and hyperglycemia >300 mg/dL
   • Recurrent diabetic ketoacidosis without precipitating infection or trauma
   • Repeated absence from work or school due to psychosocial problems causing poor metabolic control that cannot be managed as an outpatient
Severe conditions related or unrelated to diabetes that significantly affect metabolic control or are complicated by diabetes
Uncontrolled or newly discovered insulin-requiring diabetes during pregnancy
Institution of insulin-pump therapy or other intensive insulin regimens†

Adapted from: American Diabetes Association. Hospital admission guidelines for diabetes. Diabetes Care. 2004;27 Suppl 1:S103.

*Children and adolescents with newly diagnosed diabetes without severe metabolic decompensation can frequently be treated in the outpatient setting if adequate educational resources and social supports are available.

†With adequate education and supervision, intensive insulin regimens and insulin-pump therapy can be safely instituted or modified in the outpatient setting.

exception to this rule is the patient with type 2 diabetes who is at very low risk for developing ketoacidosis.)

• Tell patients to drink sugar-free liquids when hyperglycemic to prevent dehydration and help lower blood glucose levels.

• Help patients be prepared for emergencies. Provide information about sick day care (see *Sick Day Recommendations* in Chapter 2), ways to handle hyperglycemia before it occurs, and when to contact the diabetes care team about hyperglycemia (e.g., number of episodes per week, number of severe episodes).

Hypoglycemia

Because the glycemic threshold for epinephrine and glucagon production is 65 to 70 mg/dL, hypoglycemia is frequently defined as a plasma glucose level of less than 70 mg/dL. Mild hypoglycemia without significant neurologic

symptoms can generally be treated by the patient. In general, 15 g of glucose or carbohydrates will increase blood glucose 25 to 50 mg/dL. Adding protein to the acute treatment neither affects the glycemic response nor prevents subsequent hypoglycemia; adding fat may retard the absorption of glucose and actually delay the response.

One approach to avoiding "overshoot hyperglycemia" is for patients to take 15 g of carbohydrates (preferably glucose), test their blood sugar in 15 minutes, and, if necessary, take another 15 g of carbohydrates. Depending on the insulin regimen, an additional snack may be needed if they will not be eating their next meal for another 30 to 60 minutes. Examples of 15 g of carbohydrates include the foods listed below.

• 3–4 oz juice

• 4 oz regular soda

• 3 tsp jelly

• 2 tbsp (or a small box of) raisins

- 3 to 5 glucose tablets (buccal preparations are also available that allow for more rapid absorption)

- 2 tsp sugar

- 8 oz milk

If hypoglycemia is severe and the patient cannot safely ingest food because of neurologic symptoms of hypoglycemia (dizziness, weakness, loss of consciousness), another person can administer 1 mg of glucagon subcutaneously or intramuscularly to transiently increase blood glucose enough to facilitate further treatment. Remember that the effects of glucagon only last 15 to 30 minutes, so additional treatment with a snack is required. Because glucagon administration requires the assistance of others, family members or those who live with a person at risk for hypoglycemia should have appropriate training in its use. If the patient does not respond to glucagon within 15 minutes, emergency assistance is needed.

If the hypoglycemia is caused by an excess of sulfonylurea or long-acting insulin, hospitalization will likely be required because of the long half-lives of these agents. Dextrose infusion may be required to maintain normoglycemia. Rapid changes in cardiac, renal, or hepatic status may drastically alter the half-life of medications used to treat diabetes and should be evaluated as potential contributing factors.

Persons with frequent hypoglycemia often develop hypoglycemia unawareness and may not have the typical adrenergic symptoms of diaphoresis, shakiness, palpitations, nervousness, hunger, or headache. Neuroglycopenic symptoms, including irritability, difficulty concentrating, blurred vision, confusion, recall difficulty, personality changes, or seizures, may develop at lower blood sugar levels. A counter-regulatory hormone response and symptoms may return after preventing low levels for two weeks.

What do I need to tell my patients about hypoglycemia?

- Review the symptoms of hypoglycemia. Point out that they will not experience all of these symptoms but that they will generally have the same symptoms whenever they are hypoglycemic.

- Teach the "rule of 15s": Treat with 15 g of carbohydrates, wait 15 minutes, and treat with another 15 g of carbohydrates if the blood glucose level is still too low.

- Caution patients not to overtreat a hypoglycemic episode.

- Remind patients to always wear identification for diabetes and to test their blood glucose before driving a car or engaging in exercise. The general recommendation is that the blood glucose level should be >100 mg/dL prior to exercise or driving.

- Teach patients to keep glucose tablets or another form of treatment with them at all times and to be sure to keep a form of glucose in the car, purse, briefcase, pocket, gym bag, desk drawer, and night stand.

- Make sure that patients at risk for hypoglycemia have a current prescription for glucagon and that someone around them knows how to administer it.

- Provide information about when to contact providers about hypoglycemia (e.g., number of episodes per week, number of severe episodes).

- Teach patients with hypoglycemia unawareness to recognize neuroglycopenic symptoms early. These patients should have higher targets to avoid hypoglycemia until adrenergic symptoms return.

17. Care of the Hospitalized Patient with Diabetes

Persons with diabetes have a 2- to 4-fold higher hospitalization rate than do those without diabetes. Diabetes predisposes to a number of conditions that may lead to hospitalization, including coronary artery disease, cerebrovascular disease, peripheral vascular disease, nephropathy, and infection. Poorly controlled diabetes has been associated with increased infectious complications, delayed wound healing, increased medical costs, increased length of stay, and increased mortality.

The general goals for patients with diabetes in the acute care setting are:

- Avoiding hypoglycemia or hyperglycemia
- Avoiding metabolic abnormalities, such as volume depletion or electrolyte abnormalities
- Meeting nutritional needs
- Assessing educational needs

General Principles of Care

The initial history of the patient with diabetes who is admitted to the hospital should include the following information:

- Preadmission medications for diabetes
- Home glucose monitoring results
- Outpatient diet
- Hemoglobin A1C values (if available)
- History or presence of complications from diabetes

Medical Nutrition Therapy

Nutrition during hospitalization should be individualized based on body weight, comorbidities, and expected caloric expenditure. The typical daily dietary provision during catabolic illness is 25 to 35 kcal/kg body weight. Overfeeding should be avoided because it may contribute to hyperglycemia.

Monitoring the total amount of consumed carbohydrates remains a key strategy for achieving glycemic control. Usually, patients who are eating should be provided with a meal plan that includes a consistent amount of carbohydrates and has a low glycemic index. Such plans typically provide 1500–2000 kcal/day with about 50% of calories from carbohydrates, 20% from protein, and 30% from fat. Because nutritional requirements can vary greatly, consultation with a dietitian should be considered for any hospitalized patient with diabetes, particularly those who frequently require individual adjustments (e.g., adolescents, metabolically stressed patients, patients requiring liquid diets or tube feedings, pregnant women, and geriatric patients).

Glycemic Goals

The influence of hospitalization on glucose levels is difficult to predict because many factors are involved (**Table 17-1**). The tendency in most patients is toward hyperglycemia or frequent fluctuations. Inpatient consultation with an endocrinologist and other diabetes specialists should be considered for any patient with diabetes, particularly those with a new diagnosis of diabetes, with poorly controlled diabetes as an outpatient, with a history of not rapidly meeting glycemic goals, or with discovered educational deficiencies. Delays in consultation frequently are associated with an increased length of stay.

Critically Ill Patients

Multiple controlled studies support the use of insulin and tight glycemic control in critically ill patients. Van den Berghe and colleagues have shown a 42% risk reduction in intensive care

Table 17-1. Common Factors Affecting Glycemia during Hospitalization

Increased counter-regulatory hormones
Unpredictable oral/enteral/parenteral nutrition
• Illness/nausea
• NPO for tests
• Changing meal times
• Cycled tube feedings
• Parenteral nutrition, intravenous glucose
Inactivity
Timing of insulin injections
Medications that affect glycemia
(e.g., corticosteroids, vasopressors)

NPO = nothing by mouth.

unit mortality with intensive glycemic control. Similarly, the Diabetes Mellitus, Insulin Glucose Infusion in Acute Myocardial Infarction (DIGAMI) study showed that in patients with diabetes and acute myocardial infarction, insulin infusion followed by intensive subcutaneous administration of insulin improved long-term survival. The greatest effect was found in those not previously treated with insulin. The blood glucose goal recommended by the American College of Endocrinology (ACE) and the American Diabetes Association (ADA) for patients in intensive care is 80 to 110 mg/dL. A number of safe and effective insulin infusion protocols designed to achieve glycemic control in critically ill patients are now available, and many hospitals use a standardized protocol.

Non-Critically Ill Patients

Too few controlled trials have evaluated the benefit of degrees of glycemic control in hospitalized patients who are not critically ill or who have not had myocardial infarction. On the basis of available data, however, ACE and ADA recommend the following blood glucose targets for these patients:

• Pregnant patients: 80 to 100 mg/dL preprandial, <120 mg/dL 1 hour postprandial, <100 mg/dL during labor and delivery

• Other hospitalized patients: <110 mg/dL preprandial, <180 mg/dL at all other times

Regimen Adjustment in Non-Critically Ill Patients with Type 2 Diabetes

Patients with type 2 diabetes who have been treated with lifestyle modification alone and have a limited, noncritical acute illness typically do not need antihyperglycemic therapy when hospitalized. Nevertheless, blood glucose monitoring is warranted in these patients to avoid unrecognized hyperglycemia.

For patients who are taking oral diabetes drugs, the question often arises as to how to adjust their diabetes regimen during hospitalization. In patients who have had acute myocardial infarction, insulin infusion has been shown to improve outcomes, whereas sulfonylureas may increase mortality. In other settings, oral agents have not been systematically studied for inpatient use. Nevertheless, some general principles apply:

• Continuing many outpatient medications may be reasonable initially for patients without cardiac complication who were previously well controlled outside of the hospital and who are expected to eat after being hospitalized. Remember that the usual contraindications apply.

• Based on the patient's history, a dosage reduction of 25% to 50% should be considered for secretagogues because of the potentially more rigid hospital diet.

• Metformin should be immediately discontinued if any of the following is present: risk of hemodynamic instability, heart failure, dehydration, decreased renal perfusion, or impaired renal function; altered hepatic function; perioperative status; or planned radiocontrast studies.

• Thiazolidinediones (TZDs) may be continued unless New York Heart Association Class III or IV congestive heart failure occurs, concern for new or worsening edema arises, or abnormal results on liver function tests are found. Some physicians believe that TZDs simplify hospital medications because the agents remain effective even after discontinuation.

- Alpha-glucosidase inhibitors may be continued as long as the patient is eating regularly. However, these agents should not be continued if the patient is admitted with a gastrointestinal illness or develops gastrointestinal symptoms.

- Many of the newer injectables, such as exenatide and pramlintide, affect gastrointestinal motility and are not available on most inpatient formularies. Therefore, during hospitalization, insulin therapy is often preferred.

Oral hypoglycemic agents should be discontinued and insulin used instead for patients who are not eating. The same approach is indicated if oral intake is in doubt or unpredictable. In this setting, most physicians discontinue metformin because of increased concerns about hemodynamic instability and possible radiocontrast studies. TZDs may be continued except in the presence of liver function abnormalities, concern for new edema, or heart failure. Alpha-glucosidase inhibitors should be discontinued because they are only effective when taken with meals. Reassure patients that changes in therapy, particularly the initiation of insulin, will most likely be temporary.

Insulin and the Hospitalized Patient

Insulin requirements may increase with stress or illness or decrease with prolonged starvation, frequently returning to normal with resolution of the acute illness. Patients who take insulin as an outpatient should generally continue with insulin but may require modifications to their regimen.

When determining insulin requirements during hospitalization, recognize whether a patient can produce significant endogenous insulin. Several clinical features can help identify patients who may have severe insulin deficiency (**Table 17-2**). Patients determined to be significantly insulin deficient require basal insulin replacement at

Table 17-2. Characteristics of Patients with Potentially Severe Insulin Deficiency

Known type 1 diabetes
History of diabetic ketoacidosis
History of pancreatectomy or severe pancreatic dysfunction
Extended duration of diabetes (usually disease >10 years with insulin use >5 years)
History of metabolic instability with wide fluctuations in blood sugars

all times to avoid iatrogenic diabetic ketoacidosis. This is the case even if they are normoglycemic and not eating. In these patients, intravenous glucose at 5 to 10 g/hour is often given to limit the metabolic effects of starvation. Clear or full-liquid diets should not be sugar-free. Instead, patients should consume about 200 g of carbohydrates per day in divided amounts.

Basal insulin can be provided via any one of several strategies, including continuous subcutaneous insulin infusion or subcutaneous injections of intermediate-acting insulin (including premixed insulin) or long-acting insulin. Some of these methods may result in insulin peaks exceeding the basal requirements of the patient and could result in hypoglycemia if not timed with nutritional intake. This is especially important to remember in the hospital setting, where the patient may not have control of the timing of insulin or food delivery.

Before any insulin is prescribed, the properties of individual insulins should be reviewed (see Chapter 8, Insulin and New Injectables). Some of the most common errors during hospitalization are to give an insulin with both prandial and basal characteristics and then not to match food to the prandial peak (which leads to hypoglycemia) or only to treat with prandial insulin without basal insulin (which leads to hyperglycemia). Patients treated with a peaking intermediate insulin such as neutral protamine Hagedorn (NPH) may take a bedtime snack to diminish nocturnal hypoglycemia. Such snack choices should include complex carbohydrates and protein. Insulin dosing adjustments for patients who are designated NPO (nothing by mouth) are described in the following section (Periprocedure Management of Patients with Diabetes).

In patients eating meals with a consistent amount of carbohydrates, a fixed dosage of prandial insulin may be calculated, with a correction for pre-meal blood glucose level (see Chapter 8, Insulins and New Injectables). For patients capable of insulin self-management during hospitalization, carbohydrate counting may allow more flexibility in the meal plan.

The rapid-acting insulin analogues provide more physiologic prandial insulin kinetics than regular insulin and may even be administered immediately after eating if the amount of food the patient will eat is unclear. However, because of their very rapid peak of action, these insulins increase the risk of hypoglycemia if they are not appropriately timed with food. They should not be administered unless the planned meal is physically present in the room. On the other hand, regular insulin is more likely to lead to hypoglycemia in the setting of "stacking" of repeated doses because regular insulin has a longer duration of action. Appropriate adjustment of basal insulin based on fasting blood sugars and planned procedures will greatly decrease variability throughout the day.

Intravenous insulin is the only method of insulin delivery specifically developed for hospital use. Intravenous delivery of insulin allows for more rapid titration and does not rely on subcutaneous absorption. For these reasons, it is preferred in the perioperative period and in patients with cardiogenic shock or other critical illnesses.

Periprocedure Management of Patients with Diabetes

The preoperative evaluation of any patient with diabetes should include a cardiopulmonary risk assessment. Several cardiac risk stratification indices, such as the Eagle index for vascular surgery and the revised cardiac index, can help with this assessment.

If a patient with diabetes will be NPO for a procedure, scheduling the procedure early in the morning to facilitate medication adjustments is preferred. Blood glucose levels should be checked every 1 to 2 hours before, during, and immediately after procedures. The use of local or regional anesthesia is also preferred because it is less likely than general anesthesia to perturb glucose levels.

In patients with severe insulin deficiency (e.g., patients with type 1 diabetes), extra care must be taken to avoid iatrogenic ketosis. If subcutaneous insulin is to be continued, give one half to two thirds of the patient's usual dosage of intermediate-acting (e.g., NPH) insulin. If the patient uses a peakless analogue, such as insulin glargine, either a full dose or a dosage reduction of approximately 20% may be reasonable, depending on dietary history and prior glycemic control. Small dosages of regular or rapid-acting insulin may be given as a correction dose if blood glucose is above target. For long and complex procedures, intravenous insulin and dextrose infusions adjusted to maintain target blood glucose levels are preferred.

For patients with type 2 diabetes, blood glucose levels may improve while they are still NPO. Oral medications should be adjusted as described above. Generally, all oral diabetes medications are held the morning of surgery. If subcutaneous insulin is to be continued, give one half of the intermediate-acting insulin while patients are still NPO. Otherwise, general principles such as peakless insulin dosage adjustments and rapid-acting insulin correction are the same as those described earlier. Postoperatively, the diet should be reinstituted and advanced as rapidly as tolerated. Once the patient is eating and ready to return to the preoperative diabetes regimen, he or she should again be evaluated for contraindications.

- Metformin should not be restarted in patients with renal insufficiency, significant hepatic impairment, or heart failure.

- Secretagogues may need to be adjusted in a stepwise fashion based on oral intake and glycemic control.

Preparing for Discharge

If possible, institute the planned outpatient diabetes regimen prior to discharge to ensure adequate glycemic control and avoidance of hypoglycemia. Initiating new TZD therapy prior to discharge is not useful because clinical benefit is not seen for several weeks. Because the patient may have been on multiple regimens while hospitalized, review discharge prescriptions and dosages thoroughly. Diabetes survival skills and sick day rules should be reviewed to ensure outpatient safety.

Whenever possible, follow-up appointments should be scheduled prior to discharge, and an emergency contact number should be provided in case problems arise. Offer a referral for diabetes self-management education and medical nutrition therapy after discharge if the patient has never had these services or if changes in health status or therapy occur.

DIABETES RESOURCES

Telephone numbers:

American Diabetes Association (ADA): (800) 232-3472

American Association of Diabetes Educators (AADE): (800) 338-3633

AADE Diabetes Educator Access Line: (800) 832-6874

American Dietetic Association (Consumer Information): (800) 366-1655

Medic Alert: (800) 625-3788

General information Web sites:

American Diabetes Association (ADA)
www.diabetes.org

American Association of Diabetes Educators
www.diabeteseducator.org

National Diabetes Education Program
www.ndep.nih.gov

American Association of Clinical Endocrinologists (AACE)
www.aace.com

AACE Power of Prevention
www.powerofprevention.com

National Diabetes Information Clearinghouse (NDIC)
www.diabetes.niddk.nih.gov

American Dietetic Association
www.eatright.org

Council for the Advancement of Diabetes Research and Education
www.cadre-diabetes.org

United States Department of Health and Human Services: Agency for Healthcare Research and Quality (AHRQ), Diabetes
www.ahrq.gov/browse/diabetes.htm

American College of Physicians: ACP Diabetes Portal
http://diabetes.acponline.org

Insulin Pump Users Group Web site
www.insulin-pumpers.org

Online books and guidelines:

Joslin Diabetes Center
www.joslin.org
Home of *Joslin Diabetes Center Clinical Guidelines*
www.joslin.org/managing_your_diabetes_joslin_clinical_guidelines.asp

Yale Diabetes Center
http://info.med.yale.edu/intmed/endocrin/yale_diab_ctr.html
Home of the pocket book, *Diabetes Facts and Guidelines*

Barbara Davis Center for Childhood Diabetes
www.uchsc.edu/misc/diabetes/bdcmap.html
Home of the online books, *Understanding Diabetes: An Instruction Manual for Families on the Management of Diabetes* and *Type 1 Diabetes: Cellular, Molecular, & Clinical Immunology*
www.uchsc.edu/misc/diabetes/books.html

Endotext.org
www.endotext.org

Clinical trials information:

NIH ClinicalTrials.gov
www.clinicaltrials.gov/

Immune Tolerance Network
www.immunetolerance.org

Type 1 Diabetes TrialNet
www.diabetestrialnet.org

NIDDK Type 1 Diabetes Clinical Trial Information
www.niddk.nih.gov/fund/diabetesspecial funds/

Juvenile Diabetes Research Foundation
www.jdrf.org

American Diabetes Association
www.diabetes.org

Quality improvement programs:

National Diabetes Quality Improvement Alliance
www.nationaldiabetesalliance.org

NCQA Diabetes Physician Recognition Program
www.ncqa.org/dprp

Monofilament suppliers:

The cost of monofilaments is based on their attributes (e.g., type of handle, disposability, protective covers, and calibration) and on the number purchased.

Lower Extremity Amputation Prevention Program (LEAP): provides patient education material on foot care self-management and distributes reusable monofilaments for patient self-testing
(888) 275-4772 (Press 1 for HRSA publications and general information); www.bphc.hrsa.gov/leap

Medical Monofilament Manufacturing, LLC
(508) 746-7877; www.medicalmonofilament.com

Center for Specialized Diabetes Foot Care
(800) 543-9055; www.middelta.com

Connecticut Bioinstruments Inc.
(800) 336-1935; www.cbi-pace.com

North Coast Medical, Inc.
(800) 821-9319; www.ncmedical.com

Sensory Testing Systems
(888) 289-9293; www.sensorytestingsystems.com

Smith & Nephew, Inc.
(800) 458-8633; www.smith-nephew.com/us

Suggested Readings

Introduction—A Call to Action

The Ambulatory Care Quality Alliance Recommended Starter Set: Clinical Performance Measures for Ambulatory Care. Agency for Healthcare Research and Quality, Rockville, MD. Available at: www.ahrq.gov/qual/aqastart.htm. Accessed 3 October 2006.

Centers for Disease Control and Prevention. National diabetes fact sheet: general information and national estimates on diabetes in the United States, 2005. Atlanta, GA: U.S. Department of Health and Human Services, Centers for Disease Control and Prevention, 2005.

Saaddine JB, Cadwell B, Gregg EW, Engelgau MM, Vinicor F, Imperatore G, Narayan KM. Improvements in diabetes processes of care and intermediate outcomes: United States, 1988-2002. Ann Intern Med. 2006;144:465-74. [PMID: 16585660]

Shojania KG, Ranji SR, McDonald KM, Grimshaw JM, Sundaram V, Rushakoff RJ, et al. Effects of quality improvement strategies for type 2 diabetes on glycemic control: a meta-regression analysis. JAMA. 2006;296:427-40. [PMID: 16868301]

Zgibor JC, Songer TJ. External barriers to diabetes care: addressing personal and health systems issues. Diabetes Spectrum. 2001;14:23-28.

1. Improving the Quality of Care in Your Practice— A Team-Based Approach

Anderson RJ, Freedland KE, Clouse RE, Lustman PJ. The prevalence of comorbid depression in adults with diabetes: a meta-analysis. Diabetes Care. 2001;24:1069-78. [PMID: 11375373]

Clancy DE, Cope DW, Magruder KM, Huang P, Salter KH, Fields AW. Evaluating group visits in an uninsured or inadequately insured patient population with uncontrolled type 2 diabetes. Diabetes Educ. 2003;29:292-302. [PMID: 12728756]

McCulloch DK, Glasgow RE, Hampson SE, Wagner E. A systematic approach to diabetes management in the post-DCCT era. Diabetes Care. 1994;17:765-9. [PMID: 7924791]

Sadur CN, Moline N, Costa M, Michalik D, Mendlowitz D, Roller S, et al. Diabetes management in a health maintenance organization. Efficacy of care management using cluster visits. Diabetes Care. 1999;22:2011-7. [PMID: 10587835]

Trento M, Passera P, Tomalino M, Bajardi M, Pomero F, Allione A, et al. Group visits improve metabolic control in type 2 diabetes: a 2-year follow-up. Diabetes Care. 2001;24:995-1000. [PMID: 11375359]

Wagner EH, Grothaus LC, Sandhu N, Galvin MS, McGregor M, Artz K, et al. Chronic care clinics for diabetes in primary care: a system-wide randomized trial. Diabetes Care. 2001;24:695-700. [PMID: 11315833]

2. Patient Engagement and Self-Management

Alberti G. The DAWN (Diabetes Attitudes, Wishes and Needs) study. Practical Diabetology International. 2002;19:22-4.

Anderson RM, Funnell MM, Butler PM, Arnold MS, Fitzgerald JT, Feste CC. Patient empowerment. Results of a randomized controlled trial. Diabetes Care. 1995;18:943-9. [PMID: 7555554]

Barlow J, Wright C, Sheasby J, Turner A, Hainsworth J. Self-management approaches for people with chronic conditions: a review. Patient Educ Couns. 2002;48:177-87. [PMID: 12401421]

Dijkstra R, Braspenning J, Grol R. Empowering patients: how to implement a diabetes passport in hospital care. Patient Educ Couns. 2002;47:173-7. [PMID: 12191541]

DAFNE Study Group. Training in flexible, intensive insulin management to enable dietary freedom in people with type 1 diabetes: dose adjustment for normal eating (DAFNE) randomised controlled trial. BMJ. 2002;325:746. [PMID: 12364302]

Funnell MM, Anderson RM. Changing office practice and health care systems to facilitate diabetes self-management. Curr Diab Rep. 2003;3:127-33. [PMID: 12728638]

Funnell MM, Anderson RM. Empowerment and self-management of diabetes. Clinical Diabetes. 2004; 22:123-7.

Funnell MM, Kruger DF. Type 2 diabetes: treat to target. Nurse Pract. 2004;29:11-5, 19-23; quiz 23-5. [PMID: 14726786]

Funnell MM, Kruger DF, Spencer M. Self-management support for insulin therapy in type 2 diabetes. Diabetes Educ. 2004;30:274-80. [PMID: 15095517]

Funnell MM, Nwankwo R, Gillard ML, Anderson RM, Tang TS. Implementing an empowerment-based diabetes self-management education program. Diabetes Educ. 2005;31:53, 55-6, 61. [PMID: 15779247]

Gillard ML, Nwankwo R, Fitzgerald JT, Oh M, Musch DC, Johnson MW, et al. Informal diabetes education: impact on self-management and blood glucose control. Diabetes Educ. 2004;30:136-42. [PMID: 14999901]

Glasgow RE, Davis CL, Funnell MM, Beck A. Implementing practical interventions to support chronic illness self-management. Jt Comm J Qual Saf. 2003;29:563-74. [PMID: 14619349]

Glasgow RE, Funnell MM, Bonomi AE, Davis C, Beckham V, Wagner EH. Self-management aspects of the improving chronic illness care breakthrough series: implementation with diabetes and heart failure teams. Ann Behav Med. 2002;24:80-7. [PMID: 12054323]

Glasgow RE, Hiss RG, Anderson RM, Friedman NM, Hayward RA, Marrero DG, et al. Report of the health care delivery work group: behavioral research related to the establishment of a chronic disease model for diabetes care. Diabetes Care. 2001;24:124-30. [PMID: 11194217]

Mulcahy K, Maryniuk M, Peeples M, Peyrot M, Tomky D, Weaver T, et al. Diabetes self-management education core outcomes measures. Diabetes Educ. 2003;29:768-70, 773-84, 787-8 passim. [PMID: 14603868]

Norris SL, Engelgau MM, Narayan KM. Effectiveness of self-management training in type 2 diabetes: a systematic review of randomized controlled trials. Diabetes Care. 2001;24:561-87. [PMID: 11289485]

Norris SL, Lau J, Smith SJ, Schmid CH, Engelgau MM. Self-management education for adults with type 2 diabetes: a meta-analysis of the effect on glycemic control. Diabetes Care. 2002;25:1159-71. [PMID: 12087014]

Peyrot M, Rubin RR, Lauritzen T, Skovlund SE, Snoek FJ, Matthews DR, et al. Resistance to insulin therapy among patients and providers: results of the cross-national Diabetes Attitudes, Wishes, and Needs (DAWN) study. Diabetes Care. 2005;28:2673-9. [PMID: 16249538]

Piette JD, Glasgow RE. Education and self-monitoring of blood glucose. In: Gerstein HC, Haynes RB, eds. Evidence-based Diabetes Care. Ontario, CA: B.C. Decker, Inc.; 2001, 207-251.

Polonsky WH, Anderson BJ, Lohrer PA, Welch G, Jacobson AM, Aponte JE, et al. Assessment of diabetes-related distress. Diabetes Care. 1995;18:754-60. [PMID: 7555499]

Renders CM, Valk GD, Griffin SJ, Wagner EH, Eijk Van JT, Assendelft WJ. Interventions to improve the management of diabetes in primary care, outpatient, and community settings: a systematic review. Diabetes Care. 2001;24:1821-33. [PMID: 11574449]

Skovlund SE, Peyrot M. Lifestyle and behavior: The Diabetes Attitudes, Wishes, and Needs (DAWN) program: A new approach to improving outcomes of diabetes care. Diabetes Spectrum. 2005;18:136-42.

Testa MA, Simonson DC. Health economic benefits and quality of life during improved glycemic control in patients with type 2 diabetes mellitus: a randomized, controlled, double-blind trial. JAMA. 1998;280:1490-6. [PMID: 9809729]

Wagner EH, Grothaus LC, Sandhu N, Galvin MS, McGregor M, Artz K, et al. Chronic care clinics for diabetes in primary care: a system-wide randomized trial. Diabetes Care. 2001;24:695-700. [PMID: 11315833]

Weinger K. Group interventions: Emerging applications for diabetes care. Diabetes Spectrum. 2003; 16:86-112.

Williams GC, Zeldman A. Patient-centered diabetes self-management education. Curr Diab Rep. 2002;2:145-52. [PMID: 12647700]

3. Screening and Diagnosis of Diabetes

American Diabetes Association. Standards of medical care in diabetes—-2006. Diabetes Care. 2006;29 Suppl 1:S4-42. [PMID: 16373931]

Expert Committee on the Diagnosis and Classification of Diabetes Mellitus. Report of the expert committee on the diagnosis and classification of diabetes mellitus. Diabetes Care. 2003;26 Suppl 1:S5-20. [PMID: 12502614]

Skovlund SE, Peyrot M. Lifestyle and behavior: The Diabetes Attitudes, Wishes, and Needs (DAWN) program: A new approach to improving outcomes of diabetes care. Diabetes Spectrum. 2005; 18:136-42.

Tirosh A, Shai I, Tekes-Manova D, Israeli E, Pereg D, Shochat T, et al. Normal fasting plasma glucose levels and type 2 diabetes in young men. N Engl J Med. 2005;353:1454-62. [PMID: 16207847]

4. Preventing Diabetes

Buchanan TA, Xiang AH, Peters RK, Kjos SL, Marroquin A, Goico J, et al. Preservation of pancreatic beta-cell function and prevention of type 2 diabetes by pharmacological treatment of insulin resistance in high-risk Hispanic women. Diabetes. 2002;51:2796-803. [PMID: 12196473]

Chiasson JL. Acarbose for the prevention of diabetes, hypertension, and cardiovascular disease in subjects with impaired glucose tolerance: the Study to Prevent Non-Insulin-Dependent Diabetes Mellitus (STOP-NIDDM) Trial. Endocr Pract. 2006;12 Suppl 1:25-30. [PMID: 16627376]

Chiasson JL, Brindisi MC, Rabasa-Lhoret R. The prevention of type 2 diabetes: what is the evidence? Minerva Endocrinol. 2005;30:179-91. [PMID: 16208307]

Chiasson JL, Josse RG, Gomis R, Hanefeld M, Karasik A, Laakso M, et al. Acarbose for prevention of type 2 diabetes mellitus: the STOP-NIDDM randomised trial. Lancet. 2002;359:2072-7. [PMID: 12086760]

Fung TT, Schulze M, Manson JE, Willett WC, Hu FB. Dietary patterns, meat intake, and the risk of type 2 diabetes in women. Arch Intern Med. 2004;164:2235-40. [PMID: 15534160]

Knowler WC, Barrett-Connor E, Fowler SE, Hamman RF, Lachin JM, Walker EA, et al. Reduction in the incidence of type 2 diabetes with lifestyle intervention or metformin. N Engl J Med. 2002;346:393-403. [PMID: 11832527]

Practical guide to identification and treatment of overweight and obesity in adults. U.S. Department of Health and Human Services, Public Health Service, National Institutes of Health, National Heart, Lung, and Blood Institute. NIH Publication Number 00-4084. 2000. Available at: www.nhlbi.nih.gov/guidelines/obesity/prctgd_b.pdf. Accessed 3 October 2006.

Tuomilehto J, Lindström J, Eriksson JG, Valle TT, Hämäläinen H, Ilanne-Parikka P, et al. Prevention of type 2 diabetes mellitus by changes in lifestyle among subjects with impaired glucose tolerance. N Engl J Med. 2001;344:1343-50. [PMID: 11333990]

van Dam RM, Rimm EB, Willett WC, Stampfer MJ, Hu FB. Dietary patterns and risk for type 2 diabetes mellitus in U.S. men. Ann Intern Med. 2002;136:201-9. [PMID: 11827496]

5. Helping Patients Make Lifestyle Changes

Anderson JW, Randles KM, Kendall CW, Jenkins DJ. Carbohydrate and fiber recommendations for individuals with diabetes: a quantitative assessment and meta-analysis of the evidence. J Am Coll Nutr. 2004;23:5-17. [PMID 14963049]

6. Monitoring Glycemic Control

Briggs AL, Cornell S. Self-monitoring blood glucose (SMBG): now and the future. Journal of Pharmacy Practice. 2004;17:29-38.

GOAL AIC Team. Impact of active versus usual algorithmic titration of basal insulin and point-of-care versus laboratory measurement of HbA1c on glycemic control in patients with type 2 diabetes: the Glycemic Optimization with Algorithms and Labs at Point of Care (GOAL A1C) trial. Diabetes Care. 2006;29:1-8. [PMID: 16373887]

Miller CD, Barnes CS, Phillips LS, Ziemer DC, Gallina DL, Cook CB, et al. Rapid A1c availability improves clinical decision-making in an urban primary care clinic. Diabetes Care. 2003;26:1158-63. [PMID: 12663590]

Rizvi AA, Sanders MB. Assessment and monitoring of glycemic control in primary diabetes care: monitoring techniques, record keeping, meter downloads, tests of average glycemia, and point-of-care evaluation. J Am Acad Nurse Pract. 2006;18:11-21. [PMID: 16403208]

Saudek CD, Derr RL, Kalyani RR. Assessing glycemia in diabetes using self-monitoring blood glucose and hemoglobin A1c. JAMA. 2006;295:1688-97. [PMID: 16609091]

7. Oral Diabetes Drugs

Chiasson JL, Josse RG, Gomis R, Hanefeld M, Karasik A, Laakso M, et al. Acarbose treatment and the risk of cardiovascular disease and hypertension in patients with impaired glucose tolerance: the STOP-NIDDM trial. JAMA. 2003;290:486-94. [PMID: 12876091]

Effect of intensive blood-glucose control with metformin on complications in overweight patients with type 2 diabetes (UKPDS 34). UK Prospective Diabetes Study (UKPDS) Group. Lancet. 1998;352:854-65. [PMID: 9742977]

The effect of intensive treatment of diabetes on the development and progression of long-term complications in insulin-dependent diabetes mellitus. The Diabetes Control and Complications Trial Research Group. N Engl J Med. 1993;329:977-86. [PMID: 8366922]

Intensive blood-glucose control with sulphonylureas or insulin compared with conventional treatment and risk of complications in patients with type 2 diabetes (UKPDS 33). UK Prospective Diabetes Study (UKPDS) Group. Lancet. 1998;352:837-53. [PMID: 9742976]

Knowler WC, Barrett-Connor E, Fowler SE, Hamman RF, Lachin JM, Walker EA, et al. Reduction in the incidence of type 2 diabetes with lifestyle intervention or metformin. N Engl J Med. 2002;346:393-403. [PMID: 11832527]

Riddle MC, Rosenstock J, Gerich J; Insulin Glargine 4002 Study Investigators. The treat-to-target trail: randomized addition of glargine or human NPH insulin to oral therapy of type 2 diabetic patients. Diabetes Care. 2003;26:3080-6. [PMID: 14578243]

Turner RC, Cull CA, Frighi V, Holman RR. Glycemic control with diet, sulfonylurea, metformin, or insulin in patients with type 2 diabetes mellitus: progressive requirement for multiple therapies (UKPDS 49). UK Prospective Diabetes Study (UKPDS) Group. JAMA. 1999;281:2005-12. [PMID: 10359389]

8. Insulins and New Injectables

Chan JL, Abrahamson MJ. Pharmacological management of type 2 diabetes mellitus: rationale for rational use of insulin. Mayo Clin Proc. 2003;78:459-67. [PMID: 12683698]

Funnell MM, Kruger DF, Spencer M. Self-management support for insulin therapy in type 2 diabetes. Diabetes Educ. 2004;30:274-80. [PMID: 15095517]

Gaglia JL. The state of islet transplantation. Current Opinion in Internal Medicine. 2006;5:267-72.

Hirsch IB. Insulin analogues. N Engl J Med. 2005;352:174-83. [PMID: 15647580]

Korytkowski M. When oral agents fail: practical barriers to starting insulin. Int J Obes Relat Metab Disord. 2002;26 Suppl 3:S18-24. [PMID: 12174319]

Peyrot M, Rubin RR, Lauritzen T, Skovlund SE, Snoek FJ, Matthews DR, et al. Resistance to insulin therapy among patients and providers: results of the cross-national Diabetes Attitudes, Wishes, and Needs (DAWN) study. Diabetes Care. 2005;28:2673-9. [PMID: 16249538]

Riddle MC, Rosenstock J, Gerich J. The treat-to-target trial: randomized addition of glargine or human NPH insulin to oral therapy of type 2 diabetic patients. Diabetes Care. 2003;26:3080-6. [PMID: 14578243]

Rosenstock J, Zinman B, Murphy LJ, Clement SC, Moore P, Bowering CK, et al. Inhaled insulin improves glycemic control when substituted for or added to oral combination therapy in type 2 diabetes: a randomized, controlled trial. Ann Intern Med. 2005;143:549-58. [PMID: 16230721]

Rubin RR, Peyrot M. Psychological issues and treatments for people with diabetes. J Clin Psychol. 2001;57:457-78. [PMID: 11255202]

9. Obesity

Dansinger ML, Gleason JA, Griffith JL, Selker HP, Schaefer EJ. Comparison of the Atkins, Ornish, Weight Watchers, and Zone diets for weight loss and heart disease risk reduction: a randomized trial. JAMA. 2005;293:43-53. [PMID: 15632335]

Joslin Diabetes Center and Joslin Clinic. Clinical Nutrition Guideline for Overweight and Obese Adults with Type 2 Diabetes, Prediabetes or those at High Risk for Developing Type 2 Diabetes. 9/30/05. Available at: www.joslin.org/Files/Nutrition_ClinGuide.pdf. Accessed 3 October 2006.

Snow V, Barry P, Fitterman N, Qaseem A, Weiss K. Pharmacologic and surgical management of obesity in primary care: a clinical practice guideline from the American College of Physicians. Ann Intern Med. 2005;142:525-31. [PMID: 15809464]

10. Hyperlipidemia and Hypertension

Adler AI, Stratton IM, Neil HA, Yudkin JS, Matthews DR, Cull CA, et al. Association of systolic blood pressure with macrovascular and microvascular complications of type 2 diabetes (UKPDS 36): prospective observational study. BMJ. 2000;321:412-9. [PMID: 10938049]

Chobanian AV, Bakris GL, Black HR, Cushman WC, Green LA, Izzo JL Jr, et al. The Seventh Report of the Joint National Committee on Prevention, Detection, Evaluation, and Treatment of High Blood Pressure: the JNC 7 report (published erratum in JAMA. 2003;290:197). JAMA. 2003;289:2560-72. [PMID: 12748199]

Expert Panel on Detection, Evaluation, and Treatment of High Blood Cholesterol in Adults. Executive Summary of The Third Report of The National Cholesterol Education Program (NCEP) Expert Panel on Detection, Evaluation, and Treatment of High Blood Cholesterol In Adults (Adult Treatment Panel III). JAMA. 2001;285:2486-97. [PMID: 11368702]

Geiss LS, Rolka DB, Engelgau MM. Elevated blood pressure among U.S. adults with diabetes, 1988-1994. Am J Prev Med. 2002;22:42-8. [PMID: 11777678]

Grundy SM, Cleeman JI, Merz CN, Brewer HB Jr, Clark LT, Hunninghake DB, et al. Implications of recent clinical trials for the National Cholesterol Education Program Adult Treatment Panel III guidelines. Circulation. 2004;110:227-39. [PMID: 15249516]

Snow V, Aronson MD, Hornbake ER, Mottur-Pilson C, Weiss KB. Lipid control in the management of type 2 diabetes mellitus: a clinical practice guideline from the American College of Physicians. Ann Intern Med. 2004;140:644-9. [PMID: 15096336]

Snow V, Weiss KB, Mottur-Pilson C; Clinical Efficacy Assessment Subcommittee of the American College of Physicians. The evidence base for tight blood pressure control in the management of type 2 diabetes mellitus. Ann Intern Med. 2003;138:587-92. [PMID: 12667031]

Turnbull F, Neal B, Algert C, Chalmers J, Chapman N, Cutler J, et al. Effects of different blood pressure-lowering regimens on major cardiovascular events in individuals with and without diabetes mellitus: results of prospectively designed overviews of randomized trials. Arch Intern Med. 2005;165:1410-9. [PMID: 15983291]

Whelton PK, Barzilay J, Cushman WC, Davis BR, Iiamathi E, Kostis JB, et al. Clinical outcomes in antihypertensive treatment of type 2 diabetes, impaired fasting glucose concentration, and normoglycemia: Antihypertensive and Lipid-Lowering Treatment to Prevent Heart Attack Trial (ALLHAT). Arch Intern Med. 2005;165:1401-9. [PMID: 15983290]

11. Depression and Cognitive Dysfunction

Allen KV, Frier BM, Strachan MW. The relationship between type 2 diabetes and cognitive dysfunction: longitudinal studies and their methodological limitations. Eur J Pharmacol. 2004;490:169-75. [PMID: 15094083]

Cukierman T, Gerstein HC, Williamson JD. Cognitive decline and dementia in diabetes—systematic overview of prospective observational studies. Diabetologia. 2005;48:2460-9. [PMID: 16283246]

Egede LE. Effect of comorbid chronic diseases on prevalence and odds of depression in adults with diabetes. Psychosom Med. 2005;67:46-51. [PMID: 15673623]

Egede LE, Nietert PJ, Zheng D. Depression and all-cause and coronary heart disease mortality among adults with and without diabetes. Diabetes Care. 2005;28:1339-45. [PMID: 15920049]

Gregg EW, Narayan KMV. Type 2 diabetes and cognitive function: are cognitive impairment and dementia complications of type 2 diabetes? Clinical Geriatrics. 2000;57-58, 67, 71-72.

Katon WJ, Rutter C, Simon G, Lin EH, Ludman E, Ciechanowski P, et al. The association of comorbid depression with mortality in patients with type 2 diabetes. Diabetes Care. 2005;28:2668-72. [PMID: 16249537]

U.S. Preventive Services Task Force. Screening for depression: recommendations and rationale. Ann Intern Med. 2002;136:760-4. [PMID: 12020145]

12. Complications of Diabetes

Adler AI, Stratton IM, Neil HA, Yudkin JS, Matthews DR, Cull CA, et al. Association of systolic blood pressure with macrovascular and microvascular complications of type 2 diabetes (UKPDS 36): prospective observational study. BMJ. 2000;321:412-9. [PMID: 10938049]

ALLHAT Officers and Coordinators for the ALLHAT Collaborative Research Group. The Antihypertensive and Lipid-Lowering Treatment to Prevent Heart Attack Trial. Major outcomes in high-risk hypertensive patients randomized to angiotensin-converting enzyme inhibitor or calcium channel blocker vs diuretic: The Antihypertensive and Lipid-Lowering Treatment to Prevent Heart Attack Trial (ALLHAT). JAMA. 2002;288:2981-97. [PMID: 12479763]

American Diabetes Association. Standards of medical care in diabetes—2006. Diabetes Care. 2006;29 Suppl 1:S4-42. [PMID: 16373931]

Boulé NG, Haddad E, Kenny GP, Wells GA, Sigal RJ. Effects of exercise on glycemic control and body mass in type 2 diabetes mellitus: a meta-analysis of controlled clinical trials. JAMA. 2001;286:1218-27. [PMID: 11559268]

Boulton AJ, Vinik AI, Arezzo JC, Bril V, Feldman EL, Freeman R, et al. Diabetic neuropathies: a statement by the American Diabetes Association. Diabetes Care. 2005;28:956-62. [PMID: 15793206]

Cavallerano JD, Aiello LP, Cavallerano AA, Katalinic P, Hock K, Kirby R, et al. Nonmydriatic digital imaging alternative for annual retinal examination in persons with previously documented no or mild diabetic retinopathy. Am J Ophthalmol. 2005;140:667-73. [PMID: 16083842]

The effect of intensive treatment of diabetes on the development and progression of long-term complications in insulin-dependent diabetes mellitus. The Diabetes Control and Complications Trial Research Group. N Engl J Med. 1993;329:977-86. [PMID: 8366922]

Enzlin P, Mathieu C, Van den Bruel A, Bosteels J, Vanderschueren D, Demyttenaere K. Sexual dysfunction in women with type 1 diabetes: a controlled study. Diabetes Care. 2002;25:672-7. [PMID: 11919123]

Expert Panel on Detection, Evaluation, and Treatment of High Blood Cholesterol in Adults. Executive Summary of The Third Report of The National Cholesterol Education Program (NCEP) Expert Panel on Detection, Evaluation, And Treatment of High Blood Cholesterol In Adults (Adult Treatment Panel III). JAMA. 2001;285:2486-97. [PMID: 11368702]

Freeman R. Autonomic peripheral neuropathy. Lancet. 2005;365:1259-70. [PMID: 15811460]

Gregg EW, Gerzoff RB, Caspersen CJ, Williamson DF, Narayan KM. Relationship of walking to mortality among US adults with diabetes. Arch Intern Med. 2003;163:1440-7. [PMID: 12824093]

Haffner SM, Lehto S, Rönnemaa T, Pyörälä K, Laakso M. Mortality from coronary heart disease in subjects with type 2 diabetes and in nondiabetic subjects with and without prior myocardial infarction. N Engl J Med. 1998;339:229-34. [PMID: 9673301]

Intensive blood-glucose control with sulphonylureas or insulin compared with conventional treatment and risk of complications in patients with type 2 diabetes (UKPDS 33). UK Prospective Diabetes Study (UKPDS) Group. Lancet. 1998;352:837-53. [PMID: 9742976]

Kramer H, Molitch ME. Screening for kidney disease in adults with diabetes. Diabetes Care. 2005;28:1813-6. [PMID: 15983346]

Lue TF. Erectile dysfunction. N Engl J Med. 2000;342:1802-13. [PMID: 10853004]

Ramsey SD, Newton K, Blough D, McCulloch DK, Sandhu N, Reiber GE, et al. Incidence, outcomes, and cost of foot ulcers in patients with diabetes. Diabetes Care. 1999;22:382-7. [PMID: 10097914]

Rutherford D, Collier A. Sexual dysfunction in women with diabetes mellitus. Gynecol Endocrinol. 2005;21:189-92. [PMID: 16316838]

Salonia A, Lanzi R, Scavini M, Pontillo M, Gatti E, Petrella G, et al. Sexual function and endocrine profile in fertile women with type 1 diabetes. Diabetes Care. 2006;29:312-6. [PMID: 16443879]

Stamler J, Wentworth D, Neaton JD. Is relationship between serum cholesterol and risk of premature death from coronary heart disease continuous and graded? Findings in 356,222 primary screenees of the Multiple Risk Factor Intervention Trial (MRFIT). JAMA. 1986;256:2823-8. [PMID: 3773199]

Tight blood pressure control and risk of macrovascular and microvascular complications in type 2 diabetes: UKPDS 38. UK Prospective Diabetes Study Group. BMJ. 1998;317:703-13. [PMID: 9732337]

Vinik A. CLINICAL REVIEW: Use of antiepileptic drugs in the treatment of chronic painful diabetic neuropathy. J Clin Endocrinol Metab. 2005;90:4936-45. [PMID: 15899953]

Wilson C, Horton M, Cavallerano J, Aiello LM. Addition of primary care-based retinal imaging technology to an existing eye care professional referral program increased the rate of surveillance and treatment of diabetic retinopathy. Diabetes Care. 2005;28:318-22. [PMID: 15677786]

Writing Team for the Diabetes Control and Complications Trial/Epidemiology of Diabetes Interventions and Complications Research Group. Effect of intensive therapy on the microvascular complications of type 1 diabetes mellitus. JAMA. 2002;287:2563-9. [PMID: 12020338]

Writing Team for the Diabetes Control and Complications Trial/Epidemiology of Diabetes Interventions and Complications Research Group. Sustained effect of intensive treatment of type 1 diabetes mellitus on development and progression of diabetic nephropathy: the Epidemiology of Diabetes Interventions and Complications (EDIC) study. JAMA. 2003;290:2159-67. [PMID: 14570951]

Yudkin JS. How can we best prolong life? Benefits of coronary risk factor reduction in non-diabetic and diabetic subjects. BMJ. 1993;306:1313-8. [PMID: 8518573]

13. Diabetes in Women of Childbearing Age

American Diabetes Association. Preconception care of women with diabetes. Diabetes Care. 2004;27 Suppl 1:S76-8. [PMID: 14693933]

Joslin Diabetes Center and Diabetes Clinic. Guideline for detection and management of diabetes in pregnancy. 9/15/05. Available at www.joslin.org/Files/Gest_guide.pdf. Accessed 3 October 2006.

14. Diabetes in Elderly Patients

Brown AF, Mangione CM, Saliba D, Sarkisian CA. Guidelines for improving the care of the older person with diabetes mellitus. J Am Geriatr Soc. 2003;51:S265-80. [PMID: 12694461]

Schwartz AV, Hillier TA, Sellmeyer DE, Resnick HE, Gregg E, Ensrud KE, et al. Older women with diabetes have a higher risk of falls: a prospective study. Diabetes Care. 2002;25:1749-54. [PMID: 12351472]

Strotmeyer ES, Cauley JA, Schwartz AV, Nevitt MC, Resnick HE, Bauer DC, et al. Nontraumatic fracture risk with diabetes mellitus and impaired fasting glucose in older white and black adults: the health, aging, and body composition study. Arch Intern Med. 2005;165:1612-7. [PMID: 16043679]

Volpato S, Leveille SG, Blaum C, Fried LP, Guralnik JM. Risk factors for falls in older disabled women with diabetes: the women's health and aging study. J Gerontol A Biol Sci Med Sci. 2005;60:1539-45. [PMID: 16424285]

15. Diabetes in Specific Ethnic Groups

Carter JS, Pugh JA, Monterrosa A. Non-insulin-dependent diabetes mellitus in minorities in the United States. Ann Intern Med. 1996;125:221-32. [PMID: 8686981]

Fan T, Koro CE, Fedder DO, Bowlin SJ. Ethnic disparities and trends in glycemic control among adults with type 2 diabetes in the U.S. from 1988 to 2002. Diabetes Care. 2006;29:1924-5. [PMID: 16873805]

McNeely MJ, Boyko EJ. Type 2 diabetes prevalence in Asian Americans: results of a national health survey. Diabetes Care. 2004;27:66-9. [PMID: 14693968]

Oldroyd J, Banerjee M, Heald A, Cruickshank K. Diabetes and ethnic minorities. Postgrad Med J. 2005;81:486-90. [PMID: 16085737]

16. Emergencies in Diabetes

American Diabetes Association. Hospital admission guidelines for diabetes. Diabetes Care. 2004;27 Suppl 1:S103. [PMID: 14693939]

American Diabetes Association. Standards of medical care in diabetes—-2006. Diabetes Care. 2006;29 Suppl 1:S4-42. [PMID: 16373931]

Gaglia JL, Wyckoff J, Abrahamson MJ. Acute hyperglycemic crisis in the elderly. Med Clin North Am. 2004;88:1063-84, xii. [PMID: 15308390]

Kitabchi AE, Umpierrez GE, Murphy MB, Barrett EJ, Kreisberg RA, Malone JI, et al. Hyperglycemic crises in diabetes. Diabetes Care. 2004;27 Suppl 1:S94-102. [PMID: 14693938]

17. Care of the Hospitalized Patient with Diabetes

Clement S, Braithwaite SS, Magee MF, Ahmann A, Smith EP, Schafer RG, et al. Management of diabetes and hyperglycemia in hospitals. Diabetes Care. 2004;27:553-91. [PMID: 14747243]

Garber AJ, Moghissi ES, Bransome ED Jr, Clark NG, Clement S, Cobin RH, et al. American College of Endocrinology position statement on inpatient diabetes and metabolic control. Endocr Pract. 2004;10:77-82. [PMID: 15251626]

Malmberg K. Prospective randomised study of intensive insulin treatment on long term survival after acute myocardial infarction in patients with diabetes mellitus. DIGAMI (Diabetes Mellitus, Insulin Glucose Infusion in Acute Myocardial Infarction) Study Group. BMJ. 1997;314:1512-5. [PMID: 9169397]

van den Berghe G, Wouters P, Weekers F, Verwaest C, Bruyninckx F, Schetz M, et al. Intensive insulin therapy in the critically ill patients. N Engl J Med. 2001;345:1359-67. [PMID: 11794168]

Index

Note: Page numbers followed by f indicate figures; those followed by t indicate tables.

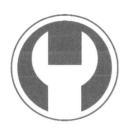

ACP
Diabetes
Care Guide
Toolkit

On the pages that follow, you will find a variety of tools that you can use to improve diabetes team care and help your patients improve their health.

You are encouraged to make copies of these tools for distribution, as the need arises. They are also provided as PDF files on the accompanying CD-ROM and on the ACP Diabetes Portal.

The tools labeled **"For Better Practice"** are for you and your staff, and the tools labeled **"For Better Health"** are for your patients.

The tools are listed in the order that they appear in the Care Guide, which explains in more detail how to incorporate the tools into your practice.

Chapter 1

For Better Practice **Assessment of Chronic Illness Care (Diabetes).** Determine where your practice is before you begin quality improvement and evaluate the effects of the changes you implement. (An easier-to-use interactive version of this tool is on the CD-ROM and the ACP Diabetes Portal at `http://diabetes.acponline.org`.)

For Better Practice **Standing Orders.** This tool will help you customize orders for patients. (An easier-to-use interactive version is on the CD-ROM and the ACP Diabetes Portal at `http://diabetes.acponline.org`.)

For Better Practice **Diabetes Care Flow Sheet**. Keep track of key examination findings for every visit.

For Better Practice **Diabetes History and Self-Management Checklist.** This tool will help you assess your patients' awareness and appreciation of many aspects of self-care.

For Better Practice **Diabetes Eye Examination Report.** Arrange to have this form completed when your patient visits the ophthalmologist.

For Better Practice **Drugs for Primary or Secondary Prevention of Cardiovascular and Kidney Disease Checklist.** This tool lists what to consider before prescribing these medications.

For Better Practice **Implementing Clinical Guidelines.** Use this tool to assign team member responsibilities to help implement clinical guidelines.

Chapter 2

For Better Health **Setting Your Self-Management Goal.** Helps patients identify goals, challenges, and strategies.

For Better Practice **Your Self-Management Workbook: Guide for Clinicians.** Guide to using the patient self-management tool *Your Self-Management Workbook* in your practice.

For Better Health **Your Self-Management Workbook.** A workbook patients can use to experiment with lifestyle changes to improve their health.

For Better Practice **Identifying Your Concerns: Guide for Clinicians.** Guide to using the *Identifying Your Concerns* questionnaire in your practice.

For Better Health **Identifying Your Concerns.** This questionnaire can help patients identify their concerns prior to their appointment.

Chapter 5

For Better Health **Rate Your Plate.** This easy-to-use tool will help patients instantly assess the nutritional value of their meals.

For Better Health **Eating Right.** Guidelines your patients can follow to eat properly.

For Better Health **Practical Exercise.** Tips that can help sedentary patients adopt a more active lifestyle.

For Better Health **Your Aerobic Exercise Plan.** A form you can use to provide patients with personalized guidelines for the aerobic exercise they have chosen.

Chapter 6

For Better Health **Monitoring Your Blood Sugar.** A checklist to help your patients monitor their blood glucose regularly.

Chapter 7

For Better Health **Keeping Track of Your Pills.** A checklist to help your patients manage their medications.

For Better Health **Your Wallet-Sized Medical Record.** A form to help your patients keep vital information handy at all times.

Chapter 8

For Better Health **Getting Started with Insulin.** Practical tips your patients can use to successfully begin insulin therapy.

Chapter 9

For Better Practice **Body Mass Index Table.** This tool will help you calculate your patients' body mass index.

Chapter 10

For Better Health **Your Diabetes Test Record.** A form for patients to record their test results and keep track of their progress.

For Better Health **The ABCs to Better Diabetes Care.** What your patients need to know about monitoring, exercise, self-management, and preventive care—on one page.

Chapter 12

For Better Practice **Sensory Foot Exam Findings.** This illustrated worksheet enables you to record the results of filament tests for 10 visits.

For Better Health **Taking Care of Your Feet.** Instructions for proper foot care that all patients with diabetes should follow.

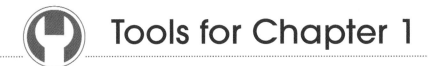

Tools for Chapter 1

For Better Practice   **Assessment of Chronic Illness Care (Diabetes)**

For Better Practice   **Standing Orders**

For Better Practice   **Diabetes Care Flow Sheet**

For Better Practice   **Diabetes History and Self-Management Checklist**

For Better Practice   **Diabetes Eye Examination Report**

For Better Practice   **Drugs for Primary or Secondary Prevention of Cardiovascular and Kidney Disease Checklist**

For Better Practice   **Implementing Clinical Guidelines**

Start improving your team care by completing this survey.

Assessment of Chronic Illness Care (Diabetes)	
Your name:	**Date:** _____/_____/_____ Month Day Year
Name of Your Practice:	Names of other persons completing the survey with you:
	1.
	2.
	3.

Directions for Using This Tool

This is a survey designed to help you move toward the "state-of-the-art" in managing chronic illnesses such as diabetes. The results can be used to help your team identify areas for improvement. Instructions are as follows:

1. **Answer each question from the perspective of one physical site** (e.g., a practice, clinic, hospital, health plan) that supports care for chronic illness.
2. **Answer each question regarding how your organization is doing** with respect to managing patients with diabetes.
3. For each row, **circle the point value** that best describes the level of care that currently exists in your practice. The rows present key aspects of chronic illness care. Each aspect is divided into levels showing various stages in improving chronic illness care. The stages are represented by points that range from 0 to 11. The higher point values indicate that the actions described in that box are more fully implemented.
4. **Total the points in each section**, calculate the average score (total score/number of questions) for each section, and enter these average scores in the space provided at the end of each section. Then add up all of the average section scores and complete the average score for the program as a whole by dividing this number by 6.

Assessment of Chronic Illness Care (Diabetes)

Part 1: Organization of the Health-Care Delivery System. Chronic illness management programs can be more effective if the overall system (organization) in which care is provided is oriented and led in a manner that allows for a focus on chronic illness care.

Components	Level D	Level C	Level B	Level A
Overall Organizational Leadership in Chronic Illness Care	...does not exist or there is a little interest.	...is reflected in vision statements and business plans, but no resources are specifically earmarked to execute the work.	...is reflected by senior leadership and specific dedicated resources (dollars and personnel).	...is part of the system's long-term planning strategy, receives necessary resources, and holds specific people accountable.
Score	0 1 2	3 4 5	6 7 8	9 10 11
Organizational Goals for Chronic Illness Care	...do not exist or are limited to one condition.	...exist but are not actively reviewed.	...are measurable and reviewed.	...are measurable, reviewed routinely, and incorporated into plans for improvement.
Score	0 1 2	3 4 5	6 7 8	9 10 11
Improvement Strategy for Chronic Illness Care	...is ad hoc and not organized or supported consistently.	...utilizes ad hoc approaches for targeted problems as they emerge.	...utilizes a proven improvement strategy for targeted problems.	...includes a proven improvement strategy and uses it proactively in meeting organizational goals.
Score	0 1 2	3 4 5	6 7 8	9 10 11
Incentives and Regulations for Chronic Illness Care	...are not used to influence clinical performance goals.	...are used to influence utilization and costs of chronic illness care.	...are used to support patient-care goals.	...are used to motivate and empower providers to support patient-care goals.
Score	0 1 2	3 4 5	6 7 8	9 10 11
Senior Leaders	...discourage enrollment of the chronically ill.	...do not make improvements to chronic illness care a priority.	...encourage improvement efforts in chronic illness care.	...visibly participate in improvement efforts in chronic illness care.
Score	0 1 2	3 4 5	6 7 8	9 10 11
Benefits	...discourage patient self-management or system changes.	...neither encourage nor discourage patient self-management or system changes.	...encourage patient self-management or system changes.	...are specifically designed to promote better chronic illness care.
Score	0 1 2	3 4 5	6 7 8	9 10 11

Total Health Care Organization Score _____ Average Score (Total Health Care Organization Score divided by 6) _____

Part 2: Community Linkages. Linkages between the health delivery system (or provider practice) and community resources play important roles in the management of chronic illness.

Components	Level D	Level C	Level B	Level A
Linking Patients to Outside Resources	...is not done systematically.	...is limited to a list of identified community resources in an accessible format.	...is accomplished through a designated staff person or resource responsible for ensuring providers and patients make maximum use of community resources.	...is accomplished through active coordination between the health system, community service agencies and patients.
Score	0 1 2	3 4 5	6 7 8	9 10 11
Partnerships with Community Organizations	...do not exist.	...are being considered but have not yet been implemented.	...are formed to develop supportive programs and policies.	...are actively sought to develop formal supportive programs and policies across the entire system.
Score	0 1 2	3 4 5	6 7 8	9 10 11
Regional Health Plans	...do not coordinate chronic illness guidelines, measures, or care resources at the practice level.	...would consider some degree of coordination of guidelines, measures, or care resources at the practice level but have not yet implemented changes.	...currently coordinate guidelines, measures, or care resources in one or two chronic illness areas.	...currently coordinate chronic illness guidelines, measures, and resources at the practice level for most chronic illnesses.
Score	0 1 2	3 4 5	6 7 8	9 10 11

Total Community Linkages Score _____ Average Score (Total Community Linkages Score divided by 3) _____

Part 3: Practice Level. Several components that manifest themselves at the level of the individual provider practice (e.g., individual clinic) have been shown to improve chronic illness care. These characteristics fall into general areas of self-management support and delivery system design issues that directly affect the practice, decision support, and clinical information systems.

Part 3a: Self-Management Support. Effective self-management support can help patients and families cope with the challenges of living with and treating chronic illness and reduce complications and symptoms.

Components	Level D	Level C	Level B	Level A
Assessment and Documentation of Self-Management Needs and Activities	...are not done.	...are expected.	...are completed in a standardized manner.	...are regularly assessed and recorded in standardized form linked to a treatment plan available to practice and patients.
Score	0 1 2	3 4 5	6 7 8	9 10 11
Self-Management Support	...is limited to distribution of information (pamphlets, booklets).	...is available by referral to self-management classes or educators.	...is provided by designated trained clinical educators who do self-management support, are affiliated with each practice, and see patients on referral.	...is provided by clinical educators who are affiliated with each practice, are trained in patient empowerment and problem-solving methodologies, and see most patients with chronic illness.
Score	0 1 2	3 4 5	6 7 8	9 10 11
Addressing Concerns of Patients and Families	...is not consistently done.	...is provided for specific patients and families through referral.	...is encouraged; peer support, groups, and mentoring programs are available.	...is an integral part of care and includes systematic assessment and routine involvement in peer support, groups, or mentoring programs.
Score	0 1 2	3 4 5	6 7 8	9 10 11
Effective Behavior Change Interventions and Peer Support	...are not available.	...are limited to the distribution of pamphlets, booklets, or other written information.	...are available only by referral to specialized centers staffed by trained personnel.	...are readily available and an integral part of routine care.
Score	0 1 2	3 4 5	6 7 8	9 10 11

Total Self-Management Score_____ Average Score (Total Self-Management Score divided by 4) _____

Part 3b: Decision Support. Effective chronic illness management programs ensure that providers have access to evidence-based information necessary to care for patients and provide decision support. This includes evidence-based practice guidelines or protocols, specialty consultation, and provider education, as well as asking patients to make provider teams aware of effective therapies.

Components	Level D	Level C	Level B	Level A
Evidence-Based Guidelines	...are not available.	...are available but not integrated into care delivery.	...are available and supported by provider education.	...are available, supported by provider education, and integrated into care through reminders and other proven provider behavior change methods.
Score	0　　1　　2	3　　4　　5	6　　7　　8	9　　10　　11
Involvement of Specialists in Improving Primary Care	...is primarily through traditional referral.	...is achieved through specialist leadership to enhance the capacity of the overall system to routinely implement guidelines.	...includes specialist leadership and designated specialists who provide primary care team training.	...includes specialist leadership and specialist involvement in improving the care of primary care patients.
Score	0　　1　　2	3　　4　　5	6　　7　　8	9　　10　　11
Provider Education for Chronic Illness Care	...is provided sporadically.	...is provided systematically through traditional methods.	...is provided using optimal methods (e.g., academic detailing).	...includes training all practice teams in chronic illness care methods, such as population-based management and self-management support.
Score	0　　1　　2	3　　4　　5	6　　7　　8	9　　10　　11
Informing Patients about Guidelines	...is not done.	...happens on request or through system publications.	...is done through specific patient education materials for each guideline.	...includes specific materials developed for patients that describe their role in achieving guideline adherence.
Score	0　　1　　2	3　　4　　5	6　　7　　8	9　　10　　11

Total Decision Support Score_____ Average Score (Total Decision Support Score divided by 4) _____

Part 3c: Delivery System Design. Evidence suggests that effective chronic illness management involves more than simply adding additional interventions to a current system focused on acute care. It may necessitate changes to the organization of practice that affect provision of care.

Components	Level D	Level C	Level B	Level A
Practice Team Functioning	...is not addressed.	...is addressed by ensuring the availability of individuals with appropriate training in key elements of chronic illness care.	...is ensured by regular team meetings to address guidelines, roles, accountability, and problems in chronic illness care.	...is ensured by teams who meet regularly and have clearly defined roles, including patient self-management education, proactive follow-up, resource coordination, and other skills in chronic illness care.
Score	0 1 2	3 4 5	6 7 8	9 10 11
Practice Team Leadership	...is not recognized locally or by the system.	...is assumed by the organization to reside in specific organizational roles.	...is ensured by the appointment of a team leader, but his/her role in chronic illness is not defined.	...is guaranteed by the appointment of a team leader who ensures that roles and responsibilities for chronic illness care are clearly defined.
Score	0 1 2	3 4 5	6 7 8	9 10 11
Appointment System	...can schedule acute care, follow-up, and preventive visits.	...ensures scheduled follow-up with chronically ill patients.	... can accommodate innovations, such as customized visit length or group visits.	...includes organization of care that facilitates a patient's seeing multiple providers in a single visit.
Score	0 1 2	3 4 5	6 7 8	9 10 11
Follow-up	...is scheduled by patients or providers in an ad hoc fashion.	...is scheduled by the practice in accordance with guidelines.	...is ensured by the practice team by monitoring patient utilization.	...is customized to patient needs, varies in intensity and methods (phone, in person, e-mail), and ensures guideline follow-up.
Score	0 1 2	3 4 5	6 7 8	9 10 11
Planned Visits for Chronic Illness Care	...are not used.	...are occasionally used for patients with complications.	...are an option for interested patients.	...are used for all patients. Include regular assessment, preventive interventions, and self-management support.
Score	0 1 2	3 4 5	6 7 8	9 10 11
Continuity of Care	...is not a priority.	...depends on written communication among primary care providers and specialists, case managers, or disease management companies.	...between primary care providers and specialists and other relevant providers is a priority but not implemented systematically.	...is a high priority, and all chronic disease interventions include active coordination between primary care, specialists, and other relevant groups.
Score	0 1 2	3 4 5	6 7 8	9 10 11

Total Delivery System Design Score_____ Average Score (Total Delivery System Design Score divided by 6) _____

Part 3d: Clinical Information Systems. Timely, useful information about individual patients and populations of patients with chronic conditions is a critical feature of effective programs, especially those that employ population-based approaches.

Components	Level D	Level C	Level B	Level A
Registry (list of patients with specific conditions)	...is not available.	...includes name, diagnosis, contact information, and date of last contact either on paper or in a computer database.	...allows queries to sort subpopulations by clinical priorities.	...is tied to guidelines which provide prompts and reminders about needed services.
Score	0 1 2	3 4 5	6 7 8	9 10 11
Reminders to Providers	...are not available.	...include general notification of the existence of a chronic illness, but does not describe needed services at time of encounter.	...include indications of needed service for populations of patients through periodic reporting.	...include specific information for the team about guideline adherence at the time of individual patient encounters.
Score	0 1 2	3 4 5	6 7 8	9 10 11
Feedback	...is not available or is not specific to the team.	...is provided at infrequent intervals and is delivered impersonally.	...occurs at frequent enough intervals to monitor performance and is specific to the team's population.	...is timely, specific to the team, routine, and personally delivered by a respected opinion leader to improve team performance.
Score	0 1 2	3 4 5	6 7 8	9 10 11
Information about Relevant Subgroups of Patients Needing Services	...is not available.	...can only be obtained with special efforts or additional programming.	...can be obtained upon request but is not routinely available.	...is provided routinely to providers to help them deliver planned care.
Score	0 1 2	3 4 5	6 7 8	9 10 11
Patient Treatment Plans	...are not expected.	...are achieved through a standardized approach.	...are established collaboratively and include self-management and clinical goals.	...are established collaboratively and include self-management and clinical management. Follow-up occurs and guides care at every point of service.
Score	0 1 2	3 4 5	6 7 8	9 10 11

Total Clinical Information Systems Score_____ Average Score (Total Clinical Information Systems Score divided by 5) _____

Integration of Chronic Illness Care Model Components. Effective systems of care integrate and combine all elements of the Chronic Illness Care Model (e.g., by linking patients' self-management goals to information systems/registries).

Components	Little support	Basic support	Good support	Full support
Informing Patients about Guidelines	...is not done.	...happens on request or through system publications.	...is done through specific patient education materials for each guideline.	...includes specific materials developed for patients that describe their role in achieving guideline adherence.
Score	0　　1　　2	3　　4　　5	6　　7　　8	9　　10　　11
Information Systems/Registries	...do not include patient self-management goals.	...include results of patient assessments (e.g., functional status rating; readiness to engage in self-management activities), but no goals.	...include results of patient assessments and self-management goals that are developed using input from the practice team/provider and patient.	...include results of patient assessments and self-management goals that are developed using input from the practice team and patient; prompt reminders to the patient and/or provider about follow-up and periodic re-evaluation of goals.
Score	0　　1　　2	3　　4　　5	6　　7　　8	9　　10　　11
Community Programs	...do not provide feedback to the health-care system/clinic about patients' progress in their programs.	...provide sporadic feedback at joint meetings between the community and health-care system about patients' progress in their programs.	...provide regular feedback to the health-care system/clinic using formal mechanisms (e.g., Internet progress report) about patients' progress.	...provide regular feedback to the health-care system about patients' progress that requires input from patients that is then used to modify programs to better meet the needs of patients.
Score	0　　1　　2	3　　4　　5	6　　7　　8	9　　10　　11
Organizational Planning for Chronic Illness Care	...does not involve a population-based approach.	...uses data from information systems to plan care.	...uses data from information systems to proactively plan population-based care, including the development of self-management programs and partnerships with community resources.	...uses systematic data and input from practice teams to proactively plan population-based care, including the development of self-management programs and community partnerships that include a built-in evaluation plan to determine success over time.
Score	0　　1　　2	3　　4　　5	6　　7　　8	9　　10　　11
Routine Follow-up for Appointments, Patient Assessments, and Goal Planning	...is not ensured.	...is sporadically done, usually for appointments only.	...is ensured by assigning responsibilities to specific staff (e.g., nurse case manager).	...is ensured by assigning responsibilities to specific staff (e.g., nurse case manager) who use the registry and other prompts to coordinate with patients and the entire practice team.
Score	0　　1　　2	3　　4　　5	6　　7　　8	9　　10　　11
Guidelines for Chronic Illness Care	...are not shared with patients.	...are given to patients who express a specific interest in self-management of their condition.	...are provided for all patients to help them develop effective self-management or behavior modification programs and identify when they should see a provider.	...are reviewed by the practice team with the patient to devise a self-management or behavior modification program consistent with the guidelines that takes into account the patient's goals and readiness to change.
Score	0　　1　　2	3　　4　　5	6　　7　　8	9　　10　　11

Total Integration Score (Total of all scores): _____   Average Score (Total Integration Score divided by 6) = _____

(8 of 10 pages)

Briefly describe the process you used to fill out the form (e.g., reached consensus in a face-to-face meeting; filled out by the team leader in consultation with other team members, as needed; each team member filled out a separate form and the responses were averaged).

Description:

_____

_____

_____

_____

_____

_____

_____

_____

Scoring Summary

(bring forward scoring at end of each section to this page)

Total Health-Care Organization Score   _____

Total Community Linkages Score   _____

Total Self-Management Score   _____

Total Decision Support Score   _____

Total Delivery System Design Score   _____

Total Clinical Information System Score   _____

Total Integration Score   _____

Overall Total Program Score (Total of all scores)   _____

Average Program Score (Total Program divided by 7)   _____

What does it mean?

The Assessment of Chronic Illness Care (ACIC) is organized such that the highest "score" (an 11) on any individual item, subscale, or the overall score (an average of the six ACIC subscale scores) indicates optimal support for chronic illness. The lowest possible score on any given item or subscale is a 0, which corresponds to limited support for chronic illness care. The interpretation guidelines are as follows:

Between 0 and 2 = limited support for chronic illness care
Between 3 and 5 = basic support for chronic illness care
Between 6 and 8 = reasonably good support for chronic illness care
Between 9 and 11 = fully developed chronic illness care

It is fairly typical for teams to begin the collaborative program with average scores below 5 on some (or all) areas of the ACIC. After all, if everyone was providing optimal care for chronic illness, there would be no need for a chronic illness collaborative or other quality improvement programs. It is also common for teams to initially believe they are providing better care for chronic illness than they actually are. As you progress in this process, you will become more familiar with what an effective system of care involves. You may even notice your ACIC scores "declining" even though you have made improvements; this is most likely the result of your better understanding of what a good system of care looks like. Over time, as your understanding of good care increases and you continue to implement effective practice changes, you should see overall improvement on your ACIC scores.

For Better Practice: **Standing Orders**

Use this tool to customize your standing orders for patients with diabetes. Check off the tasks needed and use the associated tools identified below and included in this toolkit. An interactive version of this tool is available on your CD-ROM and at `http://diabetes.acponline.org.` *The interactive version will list only the interventions you select, providing distinct standing orders that are specific to each practice's needs.*

❑ Place *Diabetes Care Flow Sheet* (in this chapter of the toolkit) in patient record.

❑ Update *Diabetes Care Flow Sheet* with information from the patient, chart, and services rendered (below).

❑ Attach completed *Diabetes History and Self-Management Checklist* (in this chapter of the toolkit) to front of patient's chart.

❑ Administer services for every visit according to the orders below:

    ❑ Monitor and record blood pressure (on the same arm) every visit.

    ❑ Measure and record the patient's weight or body mass index every visit.

    ❑ If hemoglobin A1C value was not determined in the past 4 months, complete requisition and attach to patient's chart for physician approval.

    ❑ If a urinalysis was not done in the past year:

        ❑ Perform urine dipstick and record result in chart and flow sheet.

        ❑ If urine is negative for protein, complete a requisition for urine microalbumin measurement and attach to patient's chart for physician approval.

    ❑ If a lipid profile was not done in the past year:

        ❑ Complete a requisition for a fasting lipid profile.

        ❑ Attach the requisition to the patient's chart for physician approval.

    ❑ If a dilated eye exam was not done in the past year, complete a referral for an ophthalmology/optometry dilated eye exam and send the *Diabetes Eye Examination Report* (in this chapter of the toolkit) with the referral.

    ❑ If a foot examination was not done in the past year or if the patient complains of foot problems:

        ❑ Ask the patient to remove his or her shoes and socks.

        ❑ Perform a foot exam and record the results on the flow sheet. Foot exam to include:

❑ Palpating for the presence of dorsalis pedis and posterior tibial pulses

❑ Inspecting the skin of the feet for calluses, redness, warmth, ulcers, and ingrown toenails

❑ Using monofilament to check sensation

❑ Recording findings on the patient's flow sheet and foot chart and alerting the physician to any abnormalities

❑ Administer or arrange influenza vaccination (September through January).

❑ Document absence of contraindications to influenza vaccine, including egg allergy, previous severe reaction, acute febrile illness, previous immunization against influenza during this flu season, or patient refusal.

❑ If patient refuses vaccination, record reason for refusal in the chart.

❑ Give influenza vaccine information statement and influenza vaccine 0.5 mL, intramuscularly if > age 12 years.

❑ Record vaccine administration in the chart and the *Diabetes Care Flow Sheet.*

❑ Administer or arrange pneumococcal polysaccharide vaccine (PPV):

❑ Initial PPV administration

❑ Document absence of contraindications to the PPV, including patient refusal, or in certain circumstances, previous vaccination with PPV (see orders).

❑ If patient refuses vaccination, record reason for refusal in chart.

❑ Give PPV information statement and PPV 0.5 mL intramuscularly or subcutaneously.

❑ Record PPV administration in the chart and the *Diabetes Care Flow Sheet.*

❑ Second PPV administration

❑ Provide second dose of PPV if patient is > age 65 years and received first dose when < age 65 years but more than 5 years ago.

❑ Provide a second dose of PPV to patients who have the following conditions: damaged spleen or no spleen; sickle-cell disease; HIV or AIDS; cancer, leukemia, lymphoma, or multiple myeloma; kidney failure; nephrotic syndrome; an organ or bone marrow transplant. Also provide a second vaccine to those taking chemotherapy or long-term corticosteroids, or if more than 5 years have elapsed since first dose. If patient refuses vaccination, record reason for refusal in chart.

❑ Give PPV information statement and PPV 0.5 mL intramuscularly or subcutaneously.

❑ Record PPV administration in the chart and the *Diabetes Care Flow Sheet.*

❑ Use the *Drugs for Primary or Secondary Cardiovascular and Kidney Disease Prevention Checklist* (in this chapter of the toolkit) to identify patients who may potentially benefit from medical therapy.

❑ Attach the completed *Drugs for Primary or Secondary Prevention of Cardiovascular and Kidney Disease Checklist* to the front of the chart.

For Better Practice: **Diabetes Care Flow Sheet**

Patient name: _____

ID/Insurance #: _____

1. Record today's date in the "Dates of Service," "Dates of Results," etc., row.

2. Note compliance or record values in appropriate boxes.

History

Dates of Service						
Diabetes history and self-management history taken or updated						

(See *Diabetes History and Self-Management Checklist* in this chapter of the toolkit.)

Physical Examination

Dates of Service							
Blood pressure—every visit							
Weight—every visit							
Body mass index—every visit							
Foot examination Inspect every visit; full exam annually	Sensory (monofilament)						
	Pulses						
	Vibratory sensation						
Dilated eye exam—annually							

(See *Standing Orders* in this chapter of the toolkit.)

Laboratory Values

Dates of Results						
Hemoglobin A1C—3 times/year						
Urine microalbumin—annually						
Cholesterol—annually						
Triglycerides—annually						
HDL cholesterol—annually						
LDL cholesterol—annually						

(See *Standing Orders* in this chapter of the toolkit.)

Primary and Secondary Prevention

Date of Last Medication and Dosage							
Aspirin or other antiplatelet drug	Drug						
	Dose						
Angiotensin-converting enzyme inhibitors or angiotensin II receptor blockers	Drug						
	Dose						
Statin or other lipid-lowering drug	Drug						
	Dose						
	Drug						
	Dose						
	Drug						
	Dose						
	Drug						
	Dose						
	Drug						
	Dose						

(See *Drugs for Primary or Secondary Prevention of Cardiovascular and Kidney Disease Checklist* in this chapter of the toolkit.)

A diabetes care team member should ask a patient with diabetes the questions below and check off his or her responses. Patient education can be reinforced by providing information about goals, as needed.

Patient Name: _____

Medical Record Number: _____

The patient is: ❑ Male
                 ❑ Female

Patient age is: _____

Patient Knowledge and Reinforcement Survey:

1. "Do you know what your blood pressure should be?"   ❑ Yes
   Usual goal: Top number (systolic) <130–135;   ❑ No
   bottom number (diastolic) <80   ❑ Not sure

2. "Do you know what your cholesterol numbers should be?"
   Usual goal: LDL (bad) cholesterol <100; HDL (good)   ❑ Yes
   cholesterol >40 (men) or >50 (women); triglycerides   ❑ No
   <150. With CV risk factors, consider LDL <70.   ❑ Not sure

3. "Do you know what your hemoglobin A1C number should be?"   ❑ Yes
   Usual goal: Less than 7%   ❑ No
        ❑ Not sure

Self-Management Survey:

4. "Do you smoke?"   ❑ Yes
        ❑ No

5. "How often do you check your blood sugar (glucose) at home?"
   - ❑ Twice a day or more
   - ❑ About once a day
   - ❑ A few times a week
   - ❑ Less than once a week
   - ❑ I don't have a home glucose meter

6. "How often do you check your feet for corns, calluses, and sores?"
   - ❑ Daily or almost every day
   - ❑ A few times a week
   - ❑ Once a week
   - ❑ Twice a month
   - ❑ Monthly
   - ❑ Not at all

7. "Do you take an aspirin tablet each day?"   ❑ Yes
        ❑ No

(1 of 2 pages)

8. "Do you get a flu shot every year?" ❑ Yes
                                          ❑ No

9. "Have you ever had the pneumonia   ❑ Yes
    vaccination?"   ❑ No

10. "When was the last time you saw the eye doctor?" [   ]

11. "During a typical week, how many days do   ❑ 1 ❑ 5
    you perform at least 30 minutes of physical ❑ 2 ❑ 6
    activity that raises your heart rate?"   ❑ 3 ❑ 7
                                                 ❑ 4

Social History

12. "Many people find it hard to follow a doctor's advice or take   ❑ Yes
    all of their medications. Do you find this difficult?"   ❑ No

13. "Some people have trouble affording their medications or   ❑ Yes
    getting to their appointments. Do you find this difficult?" ❑ No

14. "Some people have other medical problems that make it   ❑ Yes
    difficult to do all the right things to keep their heart healthy, ❑ No
    such as eating a healthy diet and exercising regularly.
    Has this been a problem for you?"

15. "Some people have emotional or mental health problems that   ❑ Yes
    make it difficult to follow the doctor's recommendations or   ❑ No
    take their medications. Has this been a problem for you?"

Dietary History

16. "How many servings of fruits and vegetables do you eat   ❑ 1 ❑ 3
    in a typical day?"   ❑ 2 ❑ 4

17. "Are you currently on a low-salt (sodium-restricted) diet?" ❑ Yes
                                                                 ❑ No

18. "Are you currently on a low-fat (low-cholesterol) diet?" ❑ Yes
                                                              ❑ No

19. "Do you (or whoever buys your groceries) read the   ❑ Yes
    nutrition facts label on food items to decide whether ❑ No
    or not to buy them?"

For Better Practice: Diabetes Eye Examination Report

To:_____   **Clinic/Office:** _____

(Primary Care Provider)   **Address:** _____

Phone: _____ **Fax:** _____   _____

Patient Name :_____ **Patient ID #:** _____

Visual Acuity: _____ **R** _____ **L**   **Intraocular Pressure:** _____ **R** _____ **L**

Retinal Examination Findings:

_____ No retinopathy or past retinopathy and should be examined in one year

_____ Needs no laser now but should return in _____ months because of risk of developing diabetic macular edema (DME) or high-risk proliferative diabetic retinopathy (PDR)

_____ Diabetic macular edema requiring focal laser photocoagulation

_____ High-risk proliferative diabetic retinopathy or iris neovascularization requiring panretinal photocoagulation

_____ Tractional retinal detachment or vitreous hemorrhage requiring vitrectomy

Other Ocular Conditions

_____ Not Applicable

Cataracts:

_____ Does interfere with activities of daily living

_____ Does not interfere with activities of daily living

Glaucoma:

_____ Controlled

_____ Suboptimally controlled

Plan of Treatment:

_____ Refer to retina specialist *or:*   Follow-up in _____ weeks/months

(Check appropriate treatment plan)   *(Circle right eye "R" left eye "L" or both)*

_____ Fluorescein angiography   R   L

_____ Panretinal laser photocoagulation   R   L

_____ Focal laser photocoagulation   R   L

_____ Vitrectomy   R   L

_____ Cataract surgery   R   L

_____ Other_____

Print Name: _____   _____ _____

     Eye Care Provider (M.D. or O.D.)   Signature   Date

_____   _____ _____

Clinic/Office Name   Phone   FAX

Developed by the New Mexico Academy of Ophthalmology (www.nmao.org) and the New Mexico Medical Review Association (www.nmmra.org). Adapted with permission.

Aspirin Use Checklist

Consider prophylactic aspirin or other antiplatelet drugs in primary or secondary prevention of heart disease in patients with diabetes and no contraindications.

If the patient has any **contraindications to aspirin use**, check the appropriate box:
- ❏ Age < 18 years
- ❏ Aspirin allergy
- ❏ Peptic ulcer disease from aspirin or nonsteroidal anti-inflammatory drugs (ibuprofen, naproxen, and others)
- ❏ History of bleeding disorder
- ❏ Low platelet count

Angiotensin-Converting Enzyme (ACE) Inhibitor and Angiotensin II Receptor Blocker (ARB) Checklist

Consider use of prophylactic ACE inhibitors or ARBs (if intolerant of ACE inhibitors) in the primary or secondary prevention of heart disease in patients with diabetes who also have at least one of the following conditions:
- ❏ Hypertension
- ❏ Elevated lipid levels
- ❏ Cigarette smoking
- ❏ Microalbuminuria or proteinuria
- ❏ Previous myocardial infarction and an ejection fraction of less than 35% (by echocardiography, coronary catherization, or radionuclide imaging)

If the patient has any **contraindications to ACE inhibitor therapy**, check the appropriate box:
- ❏ Pregnancy or planning to become pregnant
- ❏ Hyperkalemia
- ❏ History of intolerable cough on ACE inhibitor therapy (may consider an ARB)
- ❏ History of angioedema on ACE inhibitor therapy

Statin or Other Lipid-Lowering Drug Checklist

Consider use of a statin or other lipid-lowering drugs in the primary or secondary prevention of heart disease in patients with diabetes and:
- ❏ LDL cholesterol > 115 mg/dL
- ❏ Any evidence of cardiovascular disease regardless of LDL cholesterol level

If the patient has any **contraindications to statin use**, check the following box:
- ❏ Previous intolerance to the drug (myalgias, rhabdomyolysis, elevated transaminase levels)

For Better Practice: Implementing Clinical Guidelines

Use this form to assign team members' responsibilities for implementing clinical guidelines.

Guideline being implemented: _____

Task	Person Responsible	When/How/Why

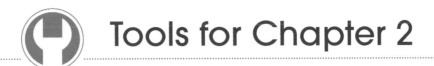

Tools for Chapter 2

For Better Health	**Setting Your Self-Management Goal**
For Better Practice	**Your Self-Management Workbook: Guide for Clinicians**
For Better Health	**Your Self-Management Workbook**
For Better Practice	**Identifying Your Concerns: Guide for Clinicians**
For Better Health	**Identifying Your Concerns**

For Better Health: **Setting Your Self-Management Goal**

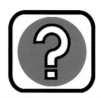 What will you do?

_____

_____

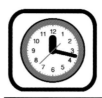 When will you do it?

_____

_____

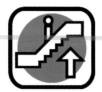 How will you do it?

_____

_____

 Where will you do it?

_____

_____

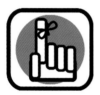 How often will you do it?

_____

_____

_____

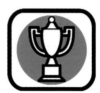 The things that could make it hard to achieve my goal are:

_____

_____

_____

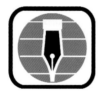 My plan for overcoming these difficulties is:

_____

_____

_____

 People who can help me achieve my goal:

_____

_____

_____

We want to **support you and help you** make your healthy change.

The best way for us to help is to hear from you about how things are going.

Contact us: _____

Follow-up instructions:

Change is Difficult
Change is Possible

- You may not succeed at first.
- You can always start over.
- Every day is a new chance to do something good for yourself.

Adapted with permission from Family Medicine Center of Akron, Summa Health System.

ACP Diabetes Care Guide • http://diabetes.acponline.org

Using *Your Self-Management Workbook* in Your Practice

Your Self-Management Workbook, the following tool in the toolkit, is designed to help patients try out lifestyle changes to improve their health. It works equally well in both one-on-one and group education settings. This workbook is based on the concept of experimenting with self-management behavior changes. It eliminates the idea of success or failure associated with achieving goals. The purpose of an experiment is to learn. Whether a plan to make a self-management change works or not, the learning associated with that experiment can be used to help the patient develop a more realistic and effective diabetes self-management plan. One way to think of *Your Self-Management Workbook* is as a continuous cycle of examining four questions with patients:

1. What does the patient want to change?

2. What did the patient try out?

3. What was the result of what the patient did?

4. What will the patient try out next?

This approach entirely eliminates the notion of success or failure, good or bad, cheating, or any of the other emotionally laden judgmental concepts that have traditionally been associated with diabetes education.

For Better Health: Your Self-Management Workbook

How to Use *Your Self-Management Workbook*

This workbook is designed to help you take steps toward better health. It is set up so that you can try out changes in your eating, physical activity, responses to stress, or other aspects of your diabetes self-management. A self-management change that fits one person's life will not necessarily fit another person's life. The final choice about what self-management plan works in your life has to be made by you.

Because it is impossible to know ahead of time which self-management changes will work for each person, this workbook has been set up as a series of experiments. The purpose of an experiment is to learn. Each time you experiment with a self-management change you learn something. You learn whether it works and whether you want to make it a permanent part of your self-management. Or you may find that it is not a change that you are willing or able to fit into your self-management plan. You can then use what you learn to plan (and try) future self-management experiments.

There is no failure in this type of program. Whether you make a change permanent or not, you know a little bit more about yourself and can make a wiser decision about your next self-management experiment.

How to Fill Out The Workbook

Following these directions you will find a sample page from the workbook followed by a page for you to fill out. In the first box, you may write down a self-management change with which you want to experiment. For example, if you want to try trading a high-fat food for a low-fat food, write that in the first box. To the right of the "Self-Management Experiment" box, write the date when you began your experiment. After trying out the new food for a number of days, you can think about how it worked and decide whether you want to make this change a regular part of your self-management plan or not. Once you decide, "Yes, I can continue with this new behavior" or "No, I cannot," you have finished the experiment. Record the date you stopped the experiment, and in the "results" box, write your conclusion from your experiment—Yes, No, Sometimes, etc. To the right of that box, write any comments you have about the experiment, such as what you learned about yourself that will help you choose your next experiment. An example of how the self-management workbook might look follows.

(1 of 3 pages)

Your Self-Management Workbook Sample Page

Self-Management Experiment	Start Date	Stop Date	Result	Comments
1. Change from whole milk to 2% milk.	2/2/2006	2/13/2006	It works.	Took a few days but tastes fine now.
2. Change from regular French dressing to reduced-calorie French dressing on salads.	2/16/2006	2/28/2006	OK.	This works fine.
3. Change from a 10-oz. steak in restaurant to a 6-oz. steak in restaurant.	3/4/2006	3/9/2006	No way!	I hate feeling hungry after a meal, especially in an expensive restaurant.
4. Trim all the fat from my steak in a restaurant.	3/9/2006	3/15/2006	Fine.	No problem.
5. Change from vegetables with margarine to vegetables plain.	3/17/2006	3/21/2006	No way!	Vegetables with all the taste sucked out.
6. Put low-fat spread on vegetables instead of margarine.	3/21/2006	3/29/2006	OK.	This ain't heaven, but I can get used to it.
7. Park in the outer lot and walk 1/4 mile to office.	4/3/2006	4/14/2006	OK.	After being late twice, I almost gave up on this one, but now that I am used to the walk, I enjoy it.
8. Walk upstairs 6 flights to cafeteria at lunch.	4/18/2006	4/26/2006	Sometimes.	I almost died the first time. Now I climb as many flights as I can and take the elevator the rest of the way.

Your Self-Management Workbook

Self-Management Experiment	Start Date	Stop Date	Result	Comments

Developed by R. M. Anderson and M. M. Funnell, Michigan Diabetes Research and Training Center. The University of Michigan. Copyright © 2005. Adapted with permission.

Using *Identifying Your Concerns* with Individual Patients

The questionnaire *Identifying Your Concerns*, the next tool in the toolkit, is designed to help you discuss with your patients their concerns regarding their diabetes. Patients should be given the opportunity to fill out the questionnaire prior to their visit or while in the waiting room. The first two questions— *"What is hardest or causing you the most concern about caring for your diabetes at this time?"* and *"Please write down a few words about what you find difficult or frustrating about the concern you mentioned above"*—serve two important functions. First, asking these questions demonstrates that you are interested in addressing the patient's primary concern (i.e., in providing patient-centered care). This approach may seem obvious, but many patients say that their visits usually begin with a discussion of test results (e.g., A1C, lipid, and blood pressure values) or that classes begin with a discussion of the definition of diabetes and that the conversation never gets around to the patients' concerns. We are not suggesting that test results be ignored but, rather, that health professionals begin visits by discussing the patient's primary concern and then address the clinical issues.

The second function that these questions serve is that they help identify the area where the patient is most likely to be motivated to make a change. Patients are not as likely to change their behavior to address the health professional's concerns (unless they are as concerned about them as the health professional) as they are to solve problems that concern them. The questions/responses below are examples of ways of helping patients describe their primary concerns:

- Summarizing example: *"Let me summarize what I've heard you say* [or wrote on the form]. *Then we can see if I've got it right."*

- *"How does this concern affect your diabetes self-care?"* Or *"How does this issue affect the rest of your life?"*

- *"What have you tried before to solve this problem and how did it work?"*

Question 3 asks, *"How would you describe your thoughts or feelings about this issue?"* Many health professionals avoid asking about feelings because they don't know how to make the patient feel better. This is a mistake. Feelings do not need to be (and usually cannot be) solved. However, feelings need to be expressed and explored for two reasons. First, the intensity of patients' feelings usually predicts the level of their motivation to make a change to improve the situation. Second, the expression of strong feelings to an empathetic listener is, in and of itself, therapeutic. Listening builds rapport. Many health professionals are surprised to learn that a study found that physician visits were on average shorter when the physician responded to patients' attempts to bring up psychosocial/emotional concerns than when the physician did not respond to such

(1 of 3 pages)

issues.[1] Below are a few examples of appropriate responses to patients' expressions of feelings:

- Empathy: *"It sounds like you have had a rough time of it."*

- Clarification: *"It sounds like you are really frustrated by your glucose readings when you are working so hard to bring them down."*

- Interest: *"How are you dealing with these feelings?"*

This is usually a good time to review what patients have circled on the assessment form. Sometimes talking about an issue results in a change in a patient's agenda. For example, patients may have indicated on the form that they didn't want to set a goal but, as result of exploring the issue, they do. Or maybe the reverse happens—they change from wanting to set a goal to not wanting to set one. If patients indicate that they do not want to set a goal at this time, ask if they wish to discuss it further that day and how you can be most helpful (e.g., talk about another issue, make a referral).

If, in response to question 4 (*"What would you like us to do during your visit to help address your concern?"*), patients indicate that they would like to come up with a plan, you may be tempted to move to setting a short-term goal quickly. However, focusing on problem-solving before the problem and the patient's emotional response to it have been explored fully is usually a mistake. Problem-solving too quickly often leads to one of two mistakes. First, if the patient and you haven't gotten to the core issue, you may end up solving the wrong problem. Second, problem-solving too quickly may prevent patients from experiencing the full intensity of their emotions, diminishing their motivation to act. When patients have had a chance to fully describe their concerns and express their feelings, it's then time to help them explore possible solutions. The following are some questions that can be used for this part of the conversation.

- *"What would have to change in order for you to feel better?"* (identifying goals)

- *"What are steps that you could take to help make things better for yourself?"*

- *"What can I do to help you?"*

- *"What will you do when you leave here?"*

To increase the probability of success, have the patient create a concrete plan. Rather than a response such as, "I guess I should talk to my husband about this," encourage the patient to create a concrete plan, such as, "I will discuss the changes I would like to make in our eating habits with my husband tonight right after he gets home from work." Plans that are concrete in terms of who, what, when, and where are much more likely to be carried out than vague, generalized plans. Inform the patient that you will ask about how the plan turned out at your next visit. This communicates interest and adds accountability. We find it useful to encourage the patient to think of their plans and short-term goals as self-management experiments. We point out that discovering what doesn't work is just as important as finding out what does work. In either case, the experiment yields new knowledge that can be used for revising the plan and conducting the next experiment. The new knowledge can also help in tailoring the self-management plan to better fit the patient. Respond to other questions and concerns as seems appropriate.

Using *Identifying Your Concerns* in Groups

Identifying Your Concerns can also be used prior to a group education program or group visit and/or incorporated into an existing assessment form. The information can then be discussed with an individual participant during the educational program or incorporated into class discussions. For example, the instructor could ask questions similar to those on the form during class and encourage the group to discuss their answers. Knowing that others have had similar experiences and feelings helps patients feel less alone with these issues.

As an alternative, the questions can be used as the basis for an interactive learning exercise during which pairs of patients discuss their answers to the assessment questions for a specific length of time (e.g., 5 minutes each). In this exercise, each patient in a pair will get to be both a speaker and a listener. For the first 5 minutes one patient presents his or her answers to the listener who asks open-ended or reflective questions to help the speaker explore and express the issues involved.

Encourage listeners to refrain from giving advice, trying to solve problems, or offering reassurance. They should encourage the expression of emotion but not try to make the speaker feel better. The job of the listener is to understand the issue from the point of view of the speaker. After 5 minutes, the patients switch roles and repeat the exercise. We often have each patient present his or her partner's issue (which encourages attentive listening during the exercise) to the entire class during the large group discussion that follows the paired sharing exercise. The two overall goals of this exercise are first, to have patients experience seeking to understand another person and second, to experience being understood by another person. Listening attentively leads to understanding. Understanding leads to acceptance. Active listening has wide applicability in everyday life.

[1]Levinson W, Gorawara-Bhat R, Lamb J. A study of patient clues and physician responses in primary care and surgical settings. JAMA 248:1021-27, 2000. [PMID: 10944650]

(3 of 3 pages)

For Better Health: Identifying Your Concerns

Please answer the following questions prior to your visit to our office. Your answers will help ensure that your concerns are addressed.

1. What is hardest or causing you the most concern about caring for your diabetes at this time? (e.g., following a diet, medication, stress)

2. Please write down a few words about what you find difficult or frustrating about the concern you mentioned above.

3. How would you describe your thoughts or feelings about this issue? (e.g., confused, angry, curious, worried, frustrated, depressed, hopeful)

4. What would you like us to do during your visit to help address your concern? (Please circle the letters in front of all expectations that apply)

    A. Work with me to come up with a plan to address this issue.

    B. I don't expect a solution. I just want you to understand what it is like for me.

    C. Refer me to another health professional or other community services.

5. I would like answers to the following questions at this visit:

6. I would like answers to these questions at some future visit:

7. Other (Please explain)

Thank you.

Developed by R. M. Anderson and M. M. Funnell, Michigan Diabetes Research and Training Center. The University of Michigan. Copyright © 2005. Adapted with permission.

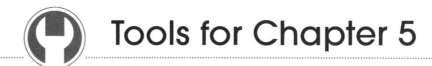

Tools for Chapter 5

For Better Health: **Rate Your Plate**

- Picture, in your mind, your usual lunch or dinner.

- Draw in lines on the plate below, and label each area for these food groups: carbohydrates, proteins, and vegetables.

Now look at the next page . . .

Does your plate look like this?

The Healthy Plate
One half vegetables, one quarter protein, one quarter carbohydrates

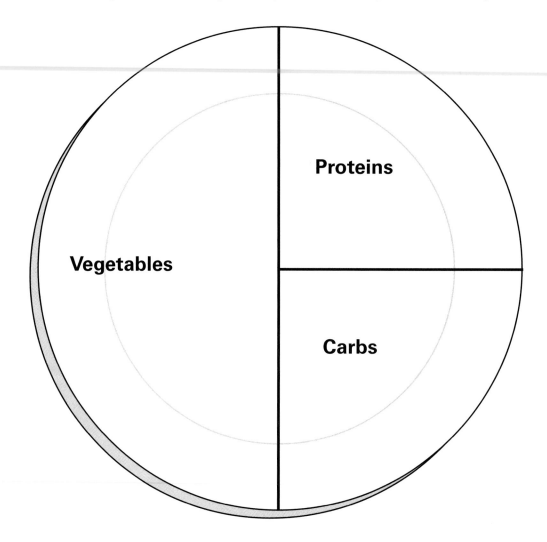

❑ Is your plate covered with colorful vegetables—dark green, orange, red, and yellow?

❑ Is the fat trimmed off your meat and the skin removed? Did you choose leaner cuts of meat, poultry, or fish?

❑ Did you choose whole grain pasta or breads? Brown rice or potato with skin?

❑ How much fat was used in cooking or added to your plate? Instead of frying, try to boil, steam, grill, or bake.

Adapted from Rate Your Plate. The Joslin Diabetes Center.

For Better Health: Eating Right

You *Can* Do It

Choose one of these easy ideas, or write down one or two things you will do for the next few weeks. Remember, little changes in your eating can make a big difference in your blood sugar.

❑ I will switch from juice or soda to diet soda.

❑ I will eat breakfast every morning.

❑ I will order regular size instead of super size at fast-food restaurants.

❑ I will pack a healthy lunch some days instead of eating out.

❑ I will keep healthy snacks on hand, like cottage cheese, carrot sticks, hard-boiled eggs, unbuttered popcorn, or sugar-free popsicles.

❑ I will eat slowly and wait before getting a second serving.

❑ _____

❑ _____

❑ _____

Adapted from Living with Diabetes: An Everyday Guide for You and Your Family. American College of Physicians Foundation. Copyright © 2006.

For Better Health: Practical Exercise

You *Can* Do It

Pick things YOU like to do. Try one of these suggestions, or write down one or two things you enjoy that make your body move.

- ❏ I will take a short walk every day.
- ❏ I will park farther away in a parking lot.
- ❏ I will dance for 20 minutes at home.
- ❏ I will get up and do small chores during television commercials.
- ❏ I will take the stairs instead of the elevator.
- ❏ I will stretch for 10 minutes when I wake up each day.
- ❏ _____
- ❏ _____

Adapted from Living with Diabetes: An Everyday Guide for You and Your Family. American College of Physicians Foundation. Copyright © 2006.

For Better Health: Your Aerobic Exercise Plan

_____   _____

Patient Name   Date

Type of Physical Activity I'd Like to Do:

❑ Walking

❑ Swimming

❑ Bicycling

❑ Stairmaster

❑ Treadmill

❑ Other: _____

Intensity:

❑ Suggested heart rate _____

❑ Perceived level of adequate exertion (able to talk in short sentences)

Duration:

• Warm up 5 to 10 minutes

• Initial duration _____ minutes   1 2 3 4 5 6 7 times per week
             (insert time)   (circle frequency)

• Goal duration _____ minutes   1 2 3 4 5 6 7 times per week
             (insert time)   (circle frequency)

_____

Physician signature

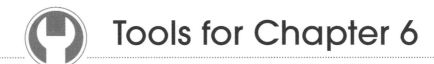 # Tools for Chapter 6

For Better Health   Monitoring Your Blood Sugar

For Better Health: Monitoring Your Blood Sugar

You *Can* Do It

Remember that you are the most important person to manage your diabetes! Choose one of these ideas, or write down one or two ways to help you take control of your blood sugar.

- ❑ I will check my blood sugar every morning, or as my doctor advises.
- ❑ I will write down my blood sugar numbers in my blood sugar log and take it to all my doctor visits.
- ❑ I will keep hard candy with me in case of an emergency.
- ❑ _____
- ❑ _____

One other thing to think about:

The A1C test

This is a blood test you get at the doctor's office. It gives your doctor an idea of what your blood sugars have been over the last 3 months. Ask your doctor what your A1C should be: _____.

Adapted from *Living with Diabetes: An Everyday Guide for You and Your Family*. American College of Physicians Foundation. Copyright © 2006.

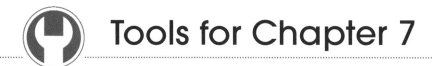

Tools for Chapter 7

You *Can* Do It

Remember, taking your pills safely can make a big difference in your blood sugar. Choose one of these easy ideas or write down one or two ways of keeping track of your pills.

❏ I will take my medicine bottles to my next doctor's appointment.

❏ I will use a pill box to help me keep track of my pills.

❏ I will ask my family to help me keep up with my pills.

❏ I will ask my pharmacist for a list of all my medicines and what they are for.

❏ I will make a list of my pills and keep it in my wallet.

❏ _____

❏ _____

For Better Health: Your Wallet-Sized Medical Record

Medical Information	Medical Information	Medical Information
Patient name:	Patient name:	Patient name:
_____	_____	_____
Doctor's name/phone:	Doctor's name/phone:	Doctor's name/phone:
_____	_____	_____
_____	_____	_____
Medical conditions	Medical conditions	Medical conditions
_____	_____	_____
_____	_____	_____
_____	_____	_____
_____	_____	_____
_____	_____	_____
Allergies	Allergies	Allergies
_____	_____	_____
_____	_____	_____
_____	_____	_____
Prescription drugs	Prescription drugs	Prescription drugs
_____	_____	_____
_____	_____	_____
_____	_____	_____
_____	_____	_____
_____	_____	_____
_____	_____	_____
_____	_____	_____
_____	_____	_____
_____	_____	_____
Over-the-counter	Over-the-counter	Over-the-counter
_____	_____	_____
_____	_____	_____
_____	_____	_____
_____	_____	_____
_____	_____	_____
Herbs/supplements	Herbs/supplements	Herbs/supplements
_____	_____	_____
_____	_____	_____
_____	_____	_____

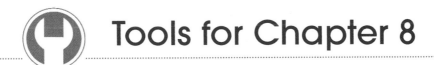

Tools for Chapter 8

For Better Health   **Getting Started with Insulin**

For Better Health: Getting Started with Insulin

You Can Do It

Remember, taking your insulin correctly makes a big difference in your blood sugar. Use these easy ideas, or write down your own ideas to make you feel more comfortable about taking insulin.

❑ I will talk with other people who take insulin shots.

❑ I will ask a friend or family member to stay with me the first few times I give myself a shot.

❑ I will practice giving shots to an orange.

❑ I will check my blood sugar before giving myself my insulin shot everyday.

❑ _____

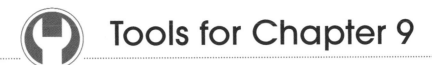

Tools for Chapter 9

For Better Practice   **Body Mass Index Table**

For Better Practice: Body Mass Index Table

BMI	Normal						Overweight					Obese										Extreme Obesity														
	19	20	21	22	23	24	25	26	27	28	29	30	31	32	33	34	35	36	37	38	39	40	41	42	43	44	45	46	47	48	49	50	51	52	53	54
Height (inches)	Body Weight (pounds)																																			
58	91	96	100	105	110	115	119	124	129	134	138	143	148	153	158	162	167	172	177	181	186	191	196	201	205	210	215	220	224	229	234	239	244	248	253	258
59	94	99	104	109	114	119	124	128	133	138	143	148	153	158	163	168	173	178	183	188	193	198	203	208	212	217	222	227	232	237	242	247	252	257	262	267
60	97	102	107	112	118	123	128	133	138	143	148	153	158	163	168	174	179	184	189	194	199	204	209	215	220	225	230	235	240	245	250	255	261	266	271	276
61	100	106	111	116	122	127	132	137	143	148	153	158	164	169	174	180	185	190	195	201	206	211	217	222	227	232	238	243	248	254	259	264	269	275	280	285
62	104	109	115	120	126	131	136	142	147	153	158	164	169	175	180	186	191	196	202	207	213	218	224	229	235	240	246	251	256	262	267	273	278	284	289	295
63	107	113	118	124	130	135	141	146	152	158	163	169	175	180	186	191	197	203	208	214	220	225	231	237	242	248	254	259	265	270	278	282	287	293	299	304
64	110	116	122	128	134	140	145	151	157	163	169	174	180	186	192	197	204	209	215	221	227	232	238	244	250	256	262	267	273	279	285	291	296	302	308	314
65	114	120	126	132	138	144	150	156	162	168	174	180	186	192	198	204	210	216	222	228	234	240	246	252	258	264	270	276	282	288	294	300	306	312	318	324
66	118	124	130	136	142	148	155	161	167	173	179	186	192	198	204	210	216	223	229	235	241	247	253	260	266	272	278	284	291	297	303	309	315	322	328	334
67	121	127	134	140	146	153	159	166	172	178	185	191	198	204	211	217	223	230	236	242	249	255	261	268	274	280	287	293	299	306	312	319	325	331	338	344
68	125	131	138	144	151	158	164	171	177	184	190	197	203	210	216	223	230	236	243	249	256	262	269	276	282	289	295	302	308	315	322	328	335	341	348	354
69	128	135	142	149	155	162	169	176	182	189	196	203	209	216	223	230	236	243	250	257	263	270	277	284	291	297	304	311	318	324	331	338	345	351	358	365
70	132	139	146	153	160	167	174	181	188	195	202	209	216	222	229	236	243	250	257	264	271	278	285	292	299	306	313	320	327	334	341	348	355	362	369	376
71	136	143	150	157	165	172	179	186	193	200	208	215	222	229	236	243	250	257	265	272	279	286	293	301	308	315	322	329	338	343	351	358	365	372	379	386
72	140	147	154	162	169	177	184	191	199	206	213	221	228	235	242	250	258	265	272	279	287	294	302	309	316	324	331	338	346	353	361	368	375	383	390	397
73	144	151	159	166	174	182	189	197	204	212	219	227	235	242	250	257	265	272	280	288	295	302	310	318	325	333	340	348	355	363	371	378	386	393	401	408
74	148	155	163	171	179	186	194	202	210	218	225	233	241	249	256	264	272	280	287	295	303	311	319	326	334	342	350	358	365	373	381	389	396	404	412	420
75	152	160	168	176	184	192	200	208	216	224	232	240	248	256	264	272	279	287	295	303	311	319	327	335	343	351	359	367	375	383	391	399	407	415	423	431
76	156	164	172	180	189	197	205	213	221	230	238	246	254	263	271	279	287	295	304	312	320	328	336	344	353	361	369	377	385	394	402	410	418	426	435	443

Reprinted from Clinical guidelines on the identification, evaluation, and treatment of overweight and obesity in adults—the evidence report. National Institutes of Health [published erratum appears in Obes Res 1998;6:464]. Obes Res. 1998;6 Suppl 2:51S-209S.

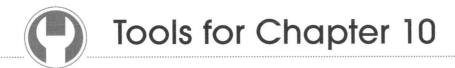

Tools for Chapter 10

For Better Health: **Your Diabetes Test Record**

Name: _____

Use this form to record your test results at each diabetes visit so you can keep track of how you are doing. The doctor, nurse, or diabetes educator will help you get started. Your doctor may add other tests to this list, such as creatinine or microalbuminuria (measures of kidney function). When you see that a test is due, mention it to the doctor or nurse to make sure that it is scheduled.

Year _____

Tests	My Goal	Date of Tests						My Notes
Weight								
Blood pressure								
A1C								
LDL								
HDL								
Triglycerides								
Eye exam								
Foot exam								

Year _____

Tests	My Goal	Date of Tests						My Notes
Weight								
Blood pressure								
A1C								
LDL								
HDL								
Triglycerides								
Eye exam								
Foot exam								

For Better Health: The ABCs to Better Diabetes Care

	How often	Ideal Level	Your Level
A1c measures blood sugar control *Lowering your A1c reduces diabetes complications*	Every 3-6 months	less than 7%	_____
Blood pressure control *Lowering your blood pressure reduces strokes*	Every visit	less than 135/80	_____
Cholesterol (LDL) level *Lowering your LDL level reduces heart attacks*	Every year	less than 100 mg/dl	_____
Diabetes kidney microalbumin test *Treating early kidney damage may prevent dialysis*	Every year	less than 30 µg/g	_____

Eye exam:
  if your last eye exam was abnormal
  if your last eye exam was normal
Detecting early eye damage may prevent blindness
	Every year
	Every 2 years		

Foot exam   ❑ observe the feet
            ❑ check pulses
            ❑ test sensation
	Every year		

Goals for self-management ❑ My goal: _____ *Helps you better control your diabetes*	Every visit		
Home glucose testing *Ask your doctor if this is right for you*	Varies		

Immunizations and Heart Medications
  ❑ Influenza (Flu vaccine)
  ❑ Pneumonia (Pneumovax)
  ❑ Statins and Aspirin - *reduce heart attacks*
Immunizations help prevent serious infections
	Every year
	At least once
	Daily if needed		

Adapted with permission from the University of Michigan Diabetes Quality Improvement Committee. The Regents of the University of Michigan. Copyright © 2006.

Tools for Chapter 12

For Better Practice: Sensory Foot Exam Findings

Put a plus sign where your patient can feel the 10-g nylon filament and a minus sign where your patient cannot feel the filament.

Date _____

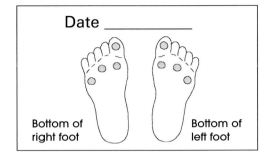

Bottom of right foot   Bottom of left foot

Date _____

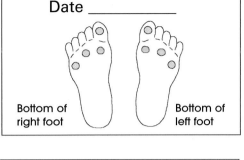

Bottom of right foot   Bottom of left foot

Date _____

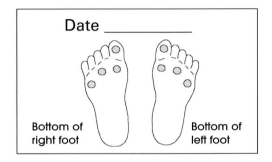

Bottom of right foot   Bottom of left foot

Date _____

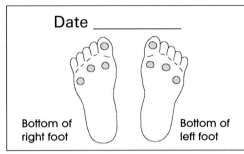

Bottom of right foot   Bottom of left foot

Date _____

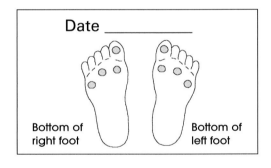

Bottom of right foot   Bottom of left foot

Date _____

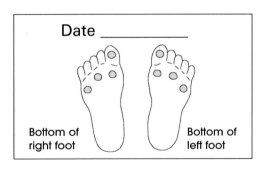

Bottom of right foot   Bottom of left foot

Date _____

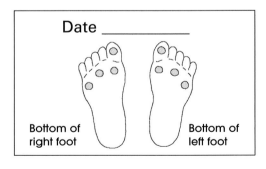

Bottom of right foot   Bottom of left foot

Date _____

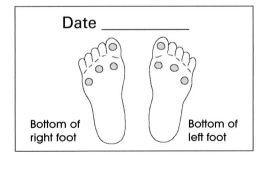

Bottom of right foot   Bottom of left foot

Date _____

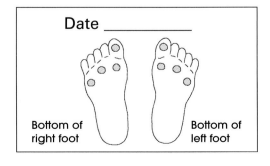

Bottom of right foot   Bottom of left foot

Date _____

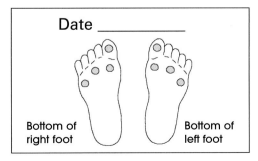

Bottom of right foot   Bottom of left foot

For Better Health: Taking Care of Your Feet

Caring for your feet is one of the simplest and most important things you can do to care for your diabetes. The two key things you can do are to look at your feet every day to make sure they have not been injured and to protect your feet from injury. Some more specific things you can do are:

Inspection

- Look at your feet each day in a place with good light. While you are drying your feet after your shower or when you take your shoes off to go to bed at night are easy times to do this.
- Look for dry places and cracks in the skin, especially between the toes and around the heel. Check for ingrown toenails, corns, calluses, blisters, red areas, swelling, or sores.
- Use a mirror if you cannot bend over to see the bottom of your feet or ask a family member for help.

Bathing

- Wash your feet in warm (not hot) water. Carefully test the water temperature with your wrist, your elbow, or a thermometer so you do not burn yourself.
- Do not soak your feet; this will dry your skin.
- Use a mild soap and rinse well. Dry your feet with a soft towel and make sure you dry between your toes.
- To soften dry feet and keep the skin from cracking, use a cream or lotion. Do not put lotion between your toes.
- If your feet sweat a lot, dust them lightly with foot powder. Wear socks that are mostly cotton, wool, or other natural fibers. Change your socks whenever they become damp or wet.

Toenails

- Trim your toenails after you bathe, when they are soft and easy to cut.
- Cut or file your nails to follow the natural curve of your toe.
- File sharp corners and rough edges of nails with an emery board so they do not cut the toes on either side.
- Do not use sharp objects to poke or dig under the toenail or around the cuticle. You can easily injure your feet with these tools.
- Ingrown toenails and nails that are thick and tend to split when cut should be cared for by a foot-care specialist.

Corns and Calluses

- After washing your feet, gently rub corns and calluses with a pumice stone to reduce buildup.
- Pad corns to reduce pressure.

(1 of 2 pages)

- Avoid over-the-counter corn or callus removers. They are harsh and can hurt healthy skin.
- Never cut your own corns and calluses with a razor blade.

Socks

- Wear soft cotton, wool, or other natural fiber socks.
- Be sure socks fit well and are not wrinkled inside of your shoes.
- Avoid socks or knee-highs with tight elastic tops, which can decrease the blood flow to your feet.

Shoes

- Choose shoes that fit well and are right for your activity for the day. Shoes that do not fit well can lead to sores, blisters, and calluses.
- Protect your feet by wearing shoes or slippers both outside and inside your house.
- Buy shoes that feel good when you first put them on and have room for all of your toes to be in their natural place. Try on shoes in the late afternoon when your feet are likely to be at their largest.
- Choose shoes with top parts that are soft and easily bent. Be sure the lining does not have ridges, wrinkles, or seams. The toe box should be round and high to allow space for all of your toes without pinching.
- To try on shoes, make an outline of each foot from stiff paper or thin cardboard. Put these into each shoe as a test of how they fit. The cardboard should not bend.
- Break in new shoes slowly by wearing them a few hours each day.
- Change your shoes at least once during the day (for example, when you come home from work).
- Before you put on your shoes, carefully check or feel for stones or rough spots that might hurt your feet.

Improve Your Blood Flow

- Begin to exercise every day.
- Avoid being in the cold for long periods of time.
- Wear warm socks.
- If you smoke, ask your doctor for help in quitting.

How to Treat Injuries

- Look at your feet for signs of an injury if you stumble or bump into something. You may not always feel pain.
- If your foot is hurt, stay off it to avoid more damage.
- Treat cuts and scratches right away. Wash with soap and water and apply a mild antiseptic. Never use strong chemicals.
- Cover the injury with a dry sterile dressing.
- Call your doctor if the sore does not begin to heal in 24 hours.

Developed by M. Ehrlich and M. M. Funnell, The University of Michigan. Copyright © 2000. Adapted with permission.

(2 of 2 pages)